GLUTEN-FREE
COMFORT FOODS

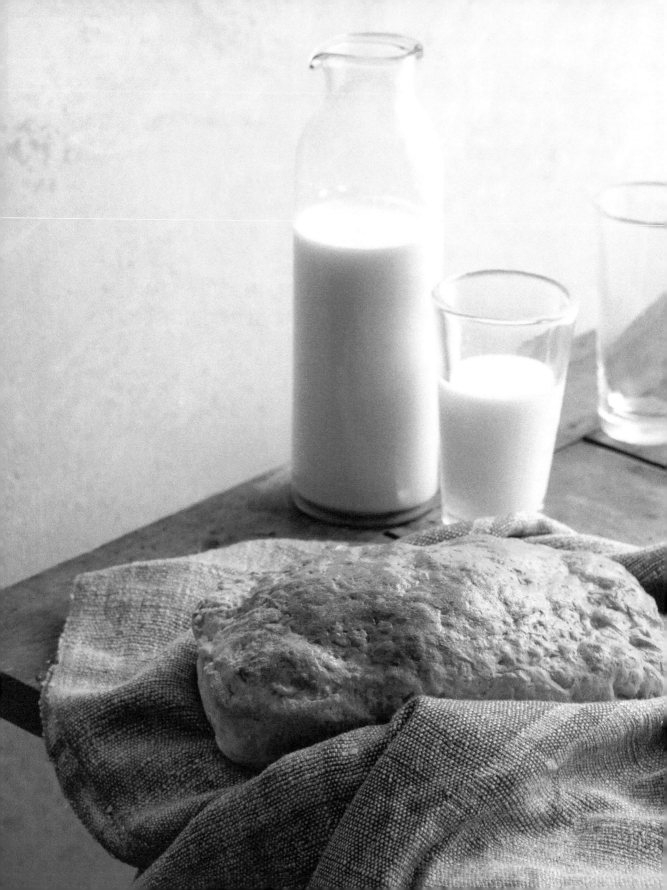

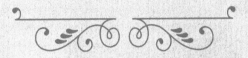

GLUTEN-FREE COMFORT FOODS

A CRAVE-WORTHY COOKBOOK
OF FAMILIAR FAVORITES

JESSICA KIRK

PHOTOGRAPHY BY ANNIE MARTIN

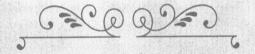

ROCKRIDGE
PRESS

Interior and Cover Designer: Angie Chiu
Art Producer: Sara Feinstein
Editor: Reina Glenn
Production Editor: Ruth Sakata Corley

Photography © 2020 Annie Martin. All other art used under license from iStock.com. Food styling by Oscar Molinar. Author photo courtesy of BlessHerHeartY'all.com

ISBN: Print 978-1-64611-890-8 | eBook 978-1-64611-891-5

R0

This book is dedicated to my father,
who taught me that life is good,
and to my mother, who taught me
to simply trust in Him.

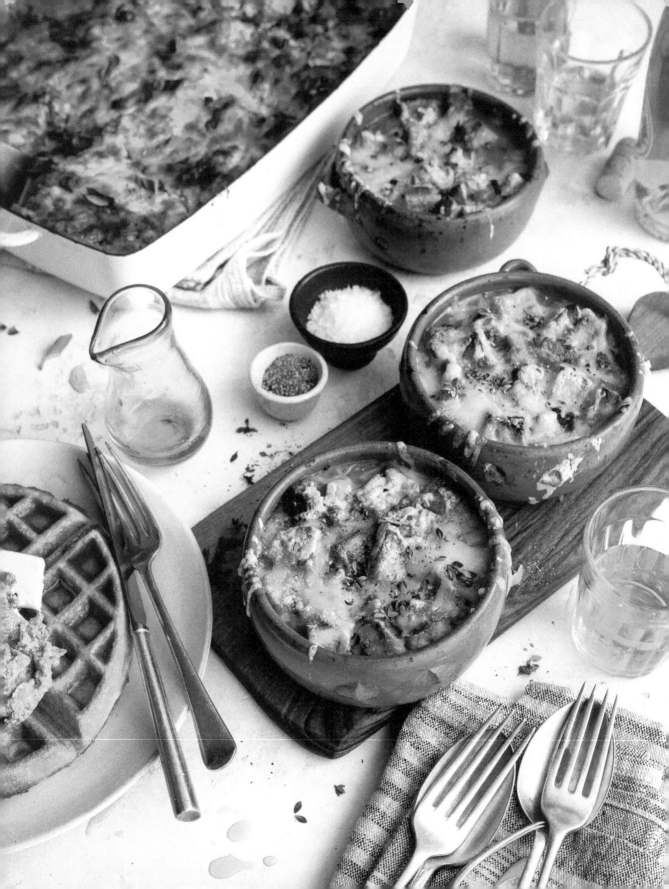

CONTENTS

INTRODUCTION

As a little girl, I would curl up in a ball and roll around the floor in pain after eating almost anything. I struggled to keep food down, became dehydrated from getting sick to my stomach, and lost large amounts of weight at a time. I was a walking skeleton. Despite countless doctors' appointments and hospital trips, no one could pinpoint what was going on.

Years later, during an emergency room visit in my early 20s, the doctor tested me for something I had never heard of: celiac disease. Sure enough, we had found the answer. Immediately, I was instructed to eliminate gluten from my diet. Problem was, a decade ago, there was next to nothing reliable to eat for people following a gluten-free lifestyle, especially when it came to comfort foods. So, after eating a lot of disappointing meals and doing a ton of research, I decided to develop my own recipes from scratch.

It took me years to create dishes I was proud of—meals full of flavor and comfort that everyone thought were delicious, even though they were gluten-free. After family members, friends, neighbors, and colleagues continuously asked me to share my recipes, I decided to start a blog. And in doing so, I encountered so many others who were dealing with the same condition. Finally, I felt like I wasn't alone.

More than six years later, I'm still running my website, Bless Her Heart Y'all, through which I've had the pleasure of swapping countless recipes, tips, tricks, and facts with my gluten-free community members, and many of my favorites made their way into this cookbook.

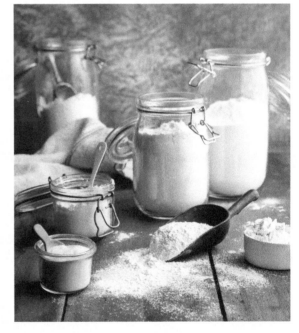

I hope this book will be a valuable resource for home cooks looking to make gluten-free comfort foods without spending a lot of time or money. Here you'll find delicious recipes, stories of my experiences (which I hope you can relate to), and a wealth of helpful tips for cooking and baking with gluten-free ingredients.

You are not alone in this journey. I am here to hold your hand and walk you through some of the things I had to learn on my own. I promise, it gets better, and this book will show you the way.

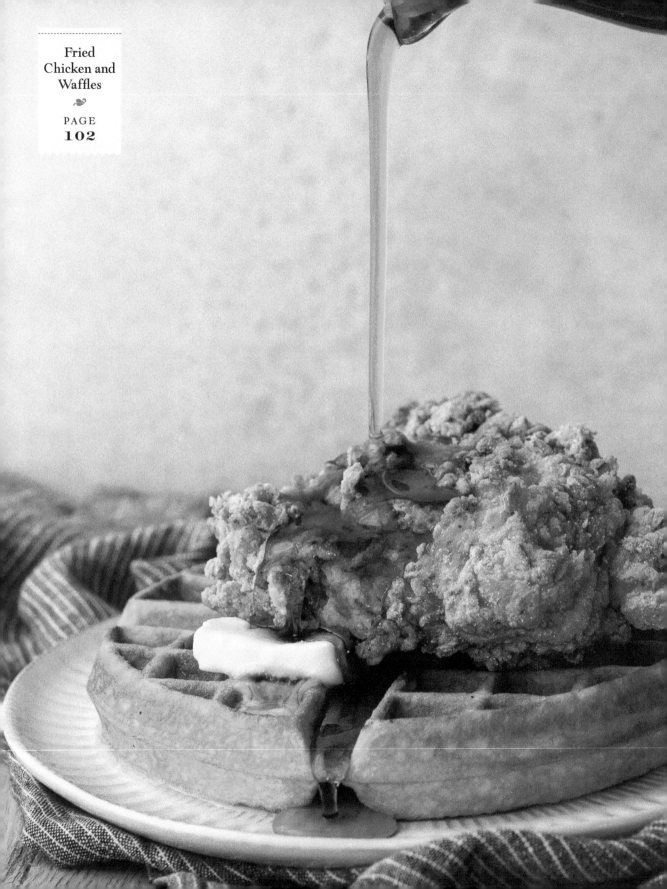

Fried
Chicken and
Waffles
❧
PAGE
102

{ 0 1 }
COMFORT FOODS GONE GLUTEN-FREE

If you're picking up this book, you may have been missing out on comfort foods for some time now. I'm happy to say that those times are about to come to an end. You no longer need to give up fluffy dinner rolls, macaroni and cheese, or your mother's hearty casserole. I'll show you how to put them back on the dinner table.

The Nostalgia of Comfort Foods

Comfort food is amazing. What else can evoke childhood memories of family, soothe that homesick feeling, and stitch together a broken heart?

Rainy days are suddenly sunny when you are homebound with the aroma of your mother's potpie. Sore throats are soothed slurping down a steaming bowl of chicken noodle soup. A stressful day at work fades after you devour a slice of chocolate cake.

Why? Because our senses bring back memories—smells, tastes, textures—that comfort foods radiate straight to our hearts. We are instantly transported. How do you feel thinking about gooey cheese stretching from slices of lasagna, warm spaghetti noodles twirling on grandma's antique fork, or that first bite of fluffy pancakes on Sunday morning?

When you're limited to a gluten-free diet, however, comfort food favorites like bread, lasagna, and pancakes may seem elusive and relegated to the past. Gluten-free diet restrictions can be daunting and very exclusionary. The good news is that today's tools and resources make it possible to bring comfort foods back onto your plate. Everyone deserves a seat at the table, including those on a gluten-free diet, so let's explore how to make it happen.

Gluten-Free Cooking at Home

Flour plays an extremely important role in cooking and baking because of a little thing called gluten. As you certainly know by now, gluten shows up in many common doughs and batters, breading for fried foods, and even thickenings for soups and gravies.

Gluten is a type of protein found in wheat, barley, and rye grains that acts as a binder. When the gluten protein reacts with liquid, it turns into a sticky substance that holds ingredients together. It's partly responsible for creating soft, doughy bites of biscuit that don't crumble and fall apart.

Without gluten, baked goods, pastas, and other flour-based recipes risk becoming brittle and fragile. You'll wind up with doughs that don't rise and cupcakes that don't fluff. Your crackers will have a rough texture, you won't have enough bounce in your biscuits, and your cookies will spread too much. And we can't let that happen.

A Guide to Gluten-Free Flours

So how do you re-create the magical effect of gluten with gluten-free ingredients? It's not as easy as replacing wheat flour with a gluten-free flour. Sometimes you need to substitute a variety of gluten-free ingredients for wheat flour. Many gluten-free home cooks turn to premade gluten-free flour mixes. Store-bought flour mixes have a place in my pantry, too, but they are pretty pricey for the small amount of flour you get and few are all they're cracked up to be.

That's why it's important to get familiar with the various gluten-free flours. You can use them on their own or in combination with each other or other gluten-free ingredients (like in my All-Purpose Flour Blend [page 171], which you can use for all the recipes in this book that call for gluten-free flour).

Here are the gluten-free flours you will see in the recipes in this book.

BROWN AND WHITE RICE FLOURS

Brown and white rice flours are made from rice and are common staples in gluten-free flours and blends. They are used in baked goods and to thicken sauces and gravies. Brown and white rice flour are integral ingredients in this book's All-Purpose Flour Blend (page 171).

TAPIOCA FLOUR

Tapioca flour is more finely ground than rice flours and has a slightly sweeter taste. It helps bind batters and creates a softer texture in doughs, just like gluten would. Tapioca flour also helps crisp up crusts and, with its touch of sweetness, is perfect for baked goods.

COCONUT FLOUR

Coconut flour is a dense, typically coarser flour. Doughs or batters that include coconut flour need to rest for at least 5 minutes to let it expand.

ALMOND FLOUR

Almond flour, used in many flour blends, is fluffy and imparts a buttery, slightly sweet flavor to baked goods. You can grind almond flour to a very fine powder, so it's perfect for when you want a smooth finish on your baked goods.

Other Gluten-Free Ingredients

Gluten-free flours often work in tandem with some sidekick ingredients that help create soft, fluffy, or stretchy textures. To truly master gluten-free cooking, you'll want to get familiar with these handy add-ins. These ingredients will likely be an initial expense, especially if you're stocking your pantry for the first time. But you'll be reusing these foundational ingredients across multiple recipes, and by following my tips for prepping in bulk, you'll maximize on your investment. You can find these products on the shelves of most retail chain grocery stores, larger health food stores, and online.

XANTHAN GUM

Xanthan gum, a powder produced from fermented simple sugars like sucrose, is one of the secret weapons of gluten-free baking. It binds liquids together, thickens sauces, and changes the texture of an otherwise crumbly baked good into a soft, fluffy one. It also provides elasticity, so your cookies will be moister and more pliable. My favorite brand is Bob's Red Mill, which you can find in most grocery store chains and health food stores. Store your xanthan gum in an airtight container so it stays fresh and can work its magic when you need it to.

CORNSTARCH

Cornstarch comes from corn and is used as a thickener in all sorts of sweet and savory recipes, gluten-free or otherwise. The recipes in this book use it for sauces, gravies, or cream-based dishes. Keep in mind that a little cornstarch goes a long way.

POTATO STARCH

Another thickener, potato starch comes from potatoes and can replace cornstarch to bulk up liquids, sauces, and gravies. It's also got a good reputation for locking in moisture, which makes it great for many gluten-free baked goods. It's another key ingredient in my All-Purpose Flour Blend (page 171).

MILK POWDER

Milk powder, or powdered milk, is the solid portion left over after milk has been dried or evaporated into a powder. Even though it's a dairy, milk powder does not need to be refrigerated, so it has a much longer shelf life than liquid milk products. Milk powder is an essential ingredient in my Biscuit Mix (page 172), offering a delightful touch of creamy sweet flavor—something many baked goods need.

Troubleshooting Common Problems

Cooking and baking with gluten-free ingredients can be tricky, especially when you are just starting out, so don't be surprised if there is a learning curve as you get comfortable, even if you're already confident in the kitchen. You'll be surprised at how many flours, gums, and powders act differently from what you're used to. Expect to run into a few hiccups while you are experimenting, such as these common gluten-free cooking issues.

Store-Bought or Homemade?

Home cooks commonly complain that store-bought gluten-free products (especially breads) are barely edible and expensive to boot. I understand this frustration. These products are unremarkable and unreliable for a number of reasons: bad flour combinations, poor-quality ingredients, failures during the mass-production process, or even poor storage techniques.

There's no way to ensure a store-bought product will be good until you take it home and try it, so I avoid the issue entirely by making my own gluten-free All-Purpose Flour Blend (page 171). I use it to make sandwich breads, cookies, pizza crusts, gravies—almost anything that requires flour. It's incredibly convenient and, because I make it in bulk, cost-effective.

Keep in mind that not every store-bought gluten-free product is awful. I have a not-so-secret list of store-bought products I've tried and loved. I don't make *everything* from scratch, and neither should you. Here's the skinny on which store-bought gluten-free products I recommend:

Pasta/noodles: Gluten-free pasta is high-quality and easy to find. I recommend Ancient Harvest corn and quinoa pastas and Barilla's gluten-free pastas. Stay away from pasta made of rice, lentils, or green vegetables, as they tend to turn to mush no matter how little you cook them.

Baking flours: Bob's Red Mill 1-to-1 Baking Flour is my go-to if I run out of my own all-purpose blend. As the name implies, it's a direct stand-in for all-purpose flour, and it works very well for most baked goods.

Soy sauce: Did you know that traditional soy sauce contains gluten? It's typically made by fermenting soybeans and crushed wheat together. My favorite gluten-free soy sauce is San-J's

Tamari Gluten-Free Soy Sauce. Or you can pick up a bottle of liquid aminos, a flavor enhancer with a taste and consistency very similar to soy sauce. If you need to steer clear of soy but still want that salty umami flavor with a slight touch of sweet, opt for a bottle of coconut aminos instead. You can swap any of these products in a 1:1 ratio.

Beer: My all-time favorite gluten-free beer is Red Bridge by Anheuser-Busch. This beer is affordable and available in many large chain grocery stores, with a moderately hoppy flavor that's not too light, not too dark. It's delicious for drinking, but I also recommend cooking with it, such as in Beer Cheese Soup (page 88).

Sausages/hot dogs: Many hot dogs and sausages have fillers and preservatives that contain wheat (and, therefore, gluten). Look for a "gluten-free" label or, even better, a "certified gluten-free" label. Alfresco brand chicken sausages are spot-on. They cook up perfectly and are easy to find in a wide variety of grocery stores. They aren't greasy, but still provide a deliciously juicy, savory flavor in every bite. As far as hot dogs go, check out Hebrew National beef franks. They are gluten-free and as good as it gets.

Chili sauce/sriracha: Many chili sauces are not categorized as gluten-free, either because of a preservative used in the recipe or because the sauce is not made in a facility that is certified gluten-free. However, there are a few delicious gluten-free options to choose from. Thai Kitchen Gluten-Free Sweet Red Chili Sauce is a very affordable option that's available in many grocery store chains and online at Target and Amazon. The best gluten-free sriracha is definitely Huy Fong's Sriracha Hot Chili Sauce, also because of its affordability and availability.

TEXTURE IS OFF

You may have heard the terms *gritty, crumbly, dense,* or *hard* used to describe gluten-free foods, or perhaps *flat, gummy,* or even *mushy*. This usually happens because you haven't replaced the gluten with the correct amount of alternative binder. Gluten holds everything together, so an unbalanced replacement can drastically change the chemistry of the finished product. This is also why you might end up with a baked good (like cookies) that spreads too much when baked.

NOT ENOUGH RISE

Gluten is responsible for the rise in traditional baked goods, which is why gluten-free home cooks sometimes end up with flat, dense treats. How do you get your baked goods to rise like they should? With a combination of things—literally. By using the right ratio of flours, starches, and add-ins, you'll be able to re-create that magical quality that makes for light, airy baked goods. This is something I tested tirelessly in developing my Sandwich Bread (page 50) and Ooey Gooey Cinnamon Rolls (page 27) recipes, both of which rise to fluffy perfection.

INCORRECT MEASUREMENTS

The super fine grind of gluten-free flours makes it hard to accurately measure them with measuring cups, which can lead to baking mishaps. Overpacking the measuring cup with flour may lead to a dense or crumbly texture, but if you don't add enough, your baked goods won't rise and they'll end up flat and sad. The trick for accurate measuring? Instead of scooping the flour straight out of the bag with the measuring cup, spoon the flour into the measuring cup until you reach the top. If you want to get even more precise, you can weigh your flour using a kitchen scale, but you'll need to convert those measurements from ounces or grams to use the recipes in this book (see the Measurement Conversions chart on page 175 for instructions).

Avoiding Cross-Contamination

As you ready your pantry for gluten-free cooking, you'll also want to remove any lingering traces of gluten. You'll have to decontaminate your kitchen on a continual basis to ensure you truly are cooking and baking gluten-free.

How do you rid your kitchen of gluten? Start by giving away or tossing the obvious forms of gluten that reside in your pantry, such as:

Breads, cookies, crackers, and pasta: Unless they already have the "gluten-free" label on their packaging, these can all go.

Condiments: Rid your kitchen of any condiments that are not gluten-free or have come into contact with products that aren't gluten-free, such as jellies, jams, and peanut butters. For example, if someone butters a piece of regular white bread and then dips the same knife into the jelly jar, the jelly is now contaminated. Double-check any open containers that could have come into contact with glutenous products for evidence, such as crumbs.

Spices: Many spices sneak gluten into their blends, so read the labels and say goodbye to anything containing wheat.

Appliances: Toasters or pans that have cooked glutenous foods should be discarded, segregated, or, at the very least, thoroughly cleaned and visually inspected to make sure no food residue remains.

If getting rid of so many things gives you heart palpitations, don't fear. At the very least, designate these items to a certain section of the kitchen or label them very well so they don't come into contact with your gluten-free cooking and baking staples.

SNEAKY PLACES YOU MIGHT FIND GLUTEN

If I had a penny for every time I found out an allegedly gluten-free food actually contained gluten, I'd be a billionaire. We know we need to avoid wheat products, but many common products have hidden gluten or traces of gluten in their ingredients, which can take the form of wheat, barley, rye, malt, or even oats. As you clean out your kitchen, keep an eye out for these possible culprits:

- **Sauces:** Such as barbecue sauce, soy sauce, and chili sauce

- **Spices and rubs:** Some spice mixes or blends contain wheat flour or wheat starch. Others may contain anticaking agents that contain gluten, such as silicon dioxide, sodium aluminum silica, and calcium silicate.

- **Tortillas:** Flour tortillas obviously contain gluten, and some brands of corn tortillas do, too.

- **Chips:** Tortilla chips, corn chips, and even potato chips may have hidden glutenous ingredients, such as wheat flour.

- **Broths and stocks:** Some broths and cooking stocks contain gluten in the form of yeast extracts made with wheat or hydro-lyzed wheat protein.

In many instances, the ingredients in products do not necessarily contain gluten, but the manufacturing plant or packaging facility may have cross-contamination issues, so the product cannot be guaranteed free from gluten. Look for the "certified gluten-free" label to be abso-lutely sure that products are guaranteed free from gluten.

Time-Saving Strategies for Gluten Freedom

You may have found that it's tough to find quality gluten-free recipes, and when you do get your hands on a great one, the time and ingre-dients called for are prohibitive. When I first started my gluten-free journey, I noticed that it took forever to work my way through gluten-free recipes because the list of ingredients was so long. I often tried to substitute my own gluten-free alternatives in traditional recipes—with varying levels of success. In this book, I've enlisted some strategies to save you a little time and effort.

LIMITED INGREDIENTS LISTS

If you've ever tried a gluten-free recipe, you may have been shocked by how many ingredients were required. Sometimes it takes three, four, even five ingredients to replicate the function that gluten plays in a certain food, and that's before you add in everything else. That's why **most recipes in this book will require 10 ingredients or fewer, and none will call for more than 14**. If I don't have the time, patience, or pocketbook for a lengthy ingredients list, I certainly don't expect you to. Keep in mind, unless a recipe states otherwise, I generally use table salt and unsalted butter, and when I use olive oil, it's regular (not extra-virgin), but feel free to use what you have on hand.

REPEATING INGREDIENTS

No one likes buying a specialty ingredient only to use 1 teaspoon and have it sit in the back of the pantry collecting dust for months to come. It's a bad use of cabinet space and it's not at all cost-effective. We'll reuse base ingredients across multiple recipes to ensure nothing goes to waste. No extra trips just to pick up one jar of spice for a single recipe.

BATCH-PREPPING

Some foods just take a while, especially baked goods. Batch-prepping allows you to create more portions of your favorite dishes for the same amount of effort, saving you time in the long run. If you make a lot at once, you'll have a dish on hand when a craving strikes. Most of the serving sizes in this book are larger than your standard four-person household because I want you to have leftovers. It's also handy if you're feeding a crowd (which comfort foods often do).

Reading the Recipes

I'm so excited for you to get started in your gluten-free kitchen. In the following pages, I'll walk you through 101 of my tried-and-true comfort food recipes.

To simplify this process even more, I have labeled each recipe with easy-to-read tags, so you know what you're getting into right from the start. Look for labels like 30 *30 Minutes or Less,* DF *Dairy-Free,* NF *Nut-Free,* and VT *Vegetarian* or V *Vegan.* You'll also notice tips at the bottom of each recipe to help guide you through the dish.

A NOTE ON DAIRY

Many readers with gluten intolerances or allergies also need to avoid dairy (myself included). While this book does not exclude dairy products, I have provided a chart of my preferred substitutions for all the types of dairy used in the recipes. There is also a substitutions chart for other common food allergies, such as eggs or nuts, on page 177. Note that changing ingredients can alter the final product's taste, texture, look, or density.

Note: Dairy products not included in the following chart but which appear in the recipes in this book include chocolate chips, Greek yogurt, sour cream, and sweetened condensed milk. I recommend replacing these ingredients with their corresponding dairy-free versions.

DAIRY INGREDIENT	REPLACE WITH	NOTES
Butter	Dairy-free butter or olive oil	Use dairy-free butter for sweets and baked goods and use olive oil for more savory dishes
Buttermilk	The liquid from a can of full-fat coconut milk mixed with lemon juice or vinegar	Mix 1 cup coconut milk liquids with 1 tablespoon lemon juice or vinegar and let stand 5 to 10 minutes before using
Cheese (all types)	Dairy-free version of the cheese in question	Some recommendations include Kite Hill Ricotta, Follow Your Heart Cheese Alternative Parmesan, and Daiya Dairy-Free Mozzarella
Cream/ Whipped cream	The liquid from a can of full-fat coconut milk or dairy-free cream	You may want to whip this before using to thicken it
Milk (whole)	Unflavored almond milk, coconut milk, or soy milk	Use coconut milk only in sweet recipes (or where you don't mind a hint of sweetness); unflavored almond and soy milks are best in savory dishes
Milk powder	Coconut milk powder	You'll only need to worry about milk powder in the recipe for the Biscuit Mix (page 172), but it's a crucial component that adds a hint of sweet creamy flavor

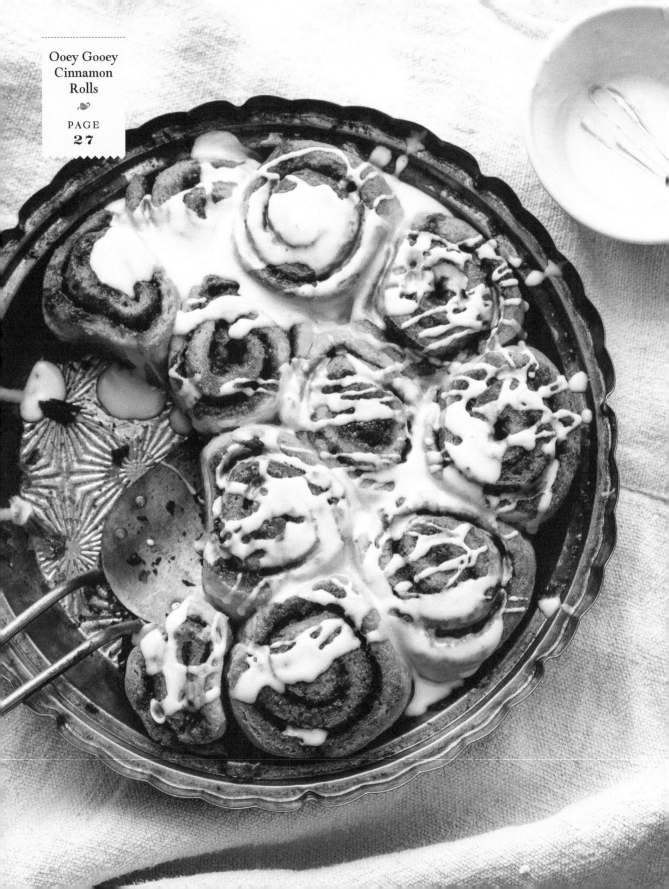

Ooey Gooey
Cinnamon
Rolls

PAGE
27

{ 0 2 }

BREAKFAST
AND BRUNCH

SWEET QUINOA BREAKFAST BARS

{ MAKES 12 BARS }

PREP TIME: 15 minutes

COOK TIME: 40 minutes

1⅓ cups water

⅔ cup uncooked gluten-free quinoa

2 large eggs

⅔ cup all-natural peanut butter

½ cup honey

1½ teaspoons gluten-free vanilla extract

⅔ cup natural applesauce

1 cup All-Purpose Flour Blend (page 171)

1 cup gluten-free oats

1 teaspoon baking soda

1½ teaspoons ground cinnamon

1¼ cups white chocolate chips, chocolate chips, dried fruit, or a combination

You're probably thinking, *What is quinoa doing in a comfort foods book?* This recipe is the perfect base for a quick, satisfying breakfast bar. Make this recipe ahead and save it for those busy mornings when it seems like you don't have enough time to get your head on straight, let alone make breakfast. It's comfort food on the go.

1. Preheat the oven to 375°F. Line a 9-by-13-inch baking pan with parchment paper.

2. In a medium saucepan, bring the water to a boil. Add the quinoa, stir, and cover. Reduce the heat to a simmer for 10 minutes, then remove from the heat and allow to sit for an additional 5 minutes, covered. Uncover, stir to fluff, and transfer to a large bowl. Refrigerate for 10 minutes to cool.

3. Add the eggs, peanut butter, honey, vanilla, and applesauce and stir. Add the flour blend, oats, baking soda, and cinnamon. Mix well to incorporate all the ingredients. Gently fold in your chocolate and fruit add-ins.

4. Pour the mixture into the pan and gently press into the bottom of the pan.

5. Bake for 18 to 22 minutes, or until the edges become golden brown.

6. Cool for 5 minutes before cutting into 12 squares and serving.

7. Store leftovers in an airtight container at room temperature for up to 1 week.

PRO TIP: Play around with the add-ins. Throw in butterscotch or caramel chips, or go a bit healthier and try dried fruits like raisins, cranberries, pineapple pieces, or dried mango bits.

MINI BLUEBERRY MUFFINS

{ MAKES 18 MINI MUFFINS }

VT 30

PREP TIME: 15 minutes

COOK TIME: 15 minutes

½ cup coconut flour

2 tablespoons coconut sugar or granulated sugar

1 teaspoon baking powder

½ teaspoon baking soda

¼ teaspoon salt

½ cup vanilla almond milk, room temperature

½ cup honey

⅓ cup coconut oil, melted

2 large eggs, room temperature

1 tablespoon apple cider vinegar

1 tablespoon unsalted butter, softened, or almond butter

1 teaspoon gluten-free vanilla extract

⅔ cup fresh blueberries

One of my favorite childhood memories is making blueberry muffins on lazy weekend mornings. My brother and I helped Dad mix the muffin batter in big bowls, attempted to fill the muffin cups (missing the mark most of the time), and tangled over who got the prized reward of licking the spoon. We devoured the little muffins in seconds, but the memories will stick with me forever.

1. Preheat the oven to 350°F. Line a mini muffin tin with muffin liners or spray with gluten-free cooking spray (see pro tip).

2. In a medium bowl, combine the coconut flour, sugar, baking powder, baking soda, and salt.

3. In a large bowl, combine the milk, honey, coconut oil, eggs, vinegar, butter, and vanilla.

4. Slowly add the dry ingredients to the wet ingredients. Using a hand mixer on low speed, mix until well combined. Allow the batter to rest for 5 minutes, until slightly thickened, then fold in the blueberries.

5. Fill each muffin cup three-quarters full with batter. Bake for 13 to 18 minutes, or until the edges are golden brown and a toothpick inserted into the center of a muffin comes out clean.

6. Cool for 5 minutes before removing the muffins from the tin, then transfer to a wire rack and cool completely before serving.

7. Store leftovers in an airtight container at room temperature for up to 3 days.

PRO TIP: This recipe will make 18 mini muffins, so use a 24-cup tin with extra room or a 12-cup pan in batches. You can use this recipe to make regular-size muffins, too. Just add 3 to 5 minutes to the baking and cooling times.

BREAKFAST BEIGNETS

{ MAKES 12 BEIGNETS }

PREP TIME: 15 minutes,
plus 1 hour to proof

COOK TIME: 15 minutes

1¾ cups All-Purpose Flour Blend
(page 171)

½ teaspoon salt

½ teaspoon xanthan gum

1 (0.75-ounce) package
instant yeast

½ cup milk

¼ cup honey

2 tablespoons unsalted
butter, softened

1 large egg, room temperature

½ teaspoon apple cider vinegar

Cooking oil, such as corn,
vegetable, or canola

1 cup powdered sugar

These pillowy clouds of dough sprinkled with
sweet powdered sugar are your morning dose of
comfort and they're so easy to make. Get your
kids involved by shaking the beignets in a bag of
sugar. A great family tradition!

1. In the bowl of a stand mixer fitted with a
   dough hook or a large bowl with a hand mixer,
   combine the flour blend, salt, and xanthan
   gum. Use your finger to poke a small hole in
   the middle of the flour mixture, then pour the
   yeast into the hole.

2. Warm the milk to around 115°F in the
   microwave, using a thermometer to check the
   temperature (it usually takes 30 to 45 seconds,
   depending on the microwave). Be careful not
   to overheat (see pro tip).

3. Pour the warm milk over the yeast, then add
   the honey, butter, egg, and vinegar. Mix until
   fully combined, about 2 minutes.

4. Cover the bowl with a clean kitchen towel and
   allow the dough to proof in a warm place for
   1 hour, or until doubled in size.

5. During the last 10 minutes of proofing, set a
   large wok or Dutch oven over medium-high
   heat and pour in 2 inches of oil. Heat the oil
   to 350°F.

6. Using a spoon, scoop out ping pong ball–size portions of dough and roll them gently into balls. Carefully drop 4 or 5 balls at a time into the hot oil. Fry for 5 minutes, flipping the balls once if they do not flip themselves, until golden brown. Use a slotted spoon to quickly scoop out the beignets, then lay them on a plate lined with paper towels. Repeat with the remaining dough. Cool until just warm to the touch, 3 to 4 minutes. (If they are too hot, the sugar coating may get soggy.)

7. Fill a paper (not plastic) bag with the powdered sugar. Once cooled, place 4 or 5 beignets inside, shake vigorously until completely coated in sugar, and remove. Repeat with the remaining beignets, and serve immediately.

8. Store leftovers in an airtight container in the refrigerator for up to 1 day. To freshen them up, toss them in a new coat of powdered sugar before serving.

PRO TIP: I recommend using a candy thermometer to test the milk temperature—if it's too cool, it won't activate the yeast; if too hot, it can kill the yeast. To test whether the oil is hot enough, drop a small bit of batter into the oil. If it sizzles immediately, the oil is ready.

EASY FLUFFY PANCAKES

{ SERVES 2 TO 4 }

PREP TIME: 5 minutes

COOK TIME: 15 minutes

3 tablespoons coconut oil

4 large eggs

¼ cup milk or heavy (whipping) cream

½ cup Biscuit Mix (page 172)

While most gluten-free pancakes are hard and dry or have a rough texture, this recipe creates soft, incredibly moist breakfast cakes to start your weekend in cozy splendor. Top with your favorite syrup, honey, or Vanilla Whipped Cream (page 169). You can even add chocolate chips to your batter for a sweet surprise.

1. In a large skillet, melt the coconut oil over low heat. Pour most of it into a large bowl, leaving a few beads of oil on the bottom of the skillet.

2. Add the eggs and milk to the large bowl and whisk until fully incorporated. Add the biscuit mix and stir until smooth.

3. Increase the heat to medium-low and spoon in ⅛ cup of batter for each pancake. Cook for 2 to 3 minutes, or until golden brown on the bottom, then flip and cook for an additional 2 to 3 minutes, until golden brown on both sides. Remove and keep warm. Repeat with the remaining batter. Serve warm.

4. Store leftovers in an airtight container in the refrigerator for up to 3 days.

CLASSIC WAFFLES

{ MAKES 3 LARGE WAFFLES }

NF VT 30

PREP TIME: 15 minutes,
plus 10 minutes to sit

COOK TIME: 15 minutes

6 large eggs

4 tablespoons unsalted
butter, melted

⅓ cup Biscuit Mix (page 172)

3 tablespoons coconut flour

1 tablespoon packed light
brown sugar

What's cozier than fluffy waffles drizzled in syrup and sprinkled with powdered sugar? These waffles take only 30 minutes to prep and cook, so not much stands between you and the breakfast of your dreams.

1. Heat a waffle maker to medium heat. If necessary, coat the inside with oil.

2. In a medium bowl, combine the eggs and butter. Use a hand mixer on low speed to mix thoroughly. Add the biscuit mix, coconut flour, and brown sugar. Mix well. Let sit for 10 minutes at room temperature.

3. Scoop ½ cup of batter onto the waffle maker, or as specified by the waffle maker instructions. Cook for about 5 minutes, until no more steam is escaping from the waffle maker and the edges of the waffle are turning golden brown. Transfer to a plate and keep warm.

4. Repeat with the remaining batter. Serve immediately (see pro tip).

5. Store leftovers in an airtight container at room temperature for up to 3 days.

PRO TIP: Top these your way. Try fresh sliced berries or banana, Vanilla Whipped Cream (page 169), nuts, powdered sugar, fresh honey, or traditional butter and maple syrup.

PERFECT BANANA BREAD

{ MAKES 1 (5-BY-9-INCH) LOAF }

PREP TIME: 10 minutes

COOK TIME: 25 minutes

1 cup sugar

2½ very ripe medium
bananas, mashed

⅔ cup brown rice flour

⅔ cup tapioca flour

⅓ cup coconut flour

⅓ cup water

⅓ cup (5⅓ tablespoons) unsalted
butter, melted

2 large eggs

1 teaspoon baking soda

½ teaspoon salt

¼ teaspoon baking powder

PRO TIP: This recipe also
makes fantastic petite bread
loaves for holiday gifting. Place
6 (3¼-by-2⅛-inch) disposable
petite loaf cups on a baking sheet
and fill them two-thirds full. Bake
at 350°F for 21 to 23 minutes, or
until the edges are golden brown
and a toothpick inserted into the
center of a loaf comes out clean.
Keep the mini loaves in their tins
when gifting.

Bananas are so fickle—you wait for days while
they ripen, then they rot in the blink of an
eye. Enter banana bread, a wonderful way to
use overly ripe bananas. This moist, cake-like
bread gives your bananas a second chance at
deliciousness. You'll never again throw away
brown bananas.

1. Preheat the oven to 350°F. Spray a 5-by-9-inch
    loaf pan with gluten-free cooking spray.

2. In a large bowl, combine the sugar, bananas,
    brown rice flour, tapioca flour, coconut flour,
    water, butter, eggs, baking soda, salt, and
    baking powder and mix well. Let stand for
    5 minutes.

3. Pour the batter into the pan (it should be about
    two-thirds full). Bake for 23 to 26 minutes, or
    until the edges of the loaf are golden brown
    and a toothpick inserted into the center of the
    loaf comes out clean.

4. Cool for 5 to 10 minutes in the pan before
    transferring to a wire rack to cool completely.
    Slice and serve.

5. Store leftovers in an airtight container at room
    temperature for up to 5 days.

GRANDMA'S OLD-FASHIONED BAKED DONUTS

{ MAKES 12 DONUTS }

PREP TIME: 10 minutes

COOK TIME: 10 minutes

FOR THE DONUTS

1¼ cups All-Purpose Flour Blend (page 171)

⅔ cup coconut sugar or granulated sugar

¼ cup flaxseed meal

1½ teaspoons baking powder

1 teaspoon xanthan gum

¼ teaspoon cream of tartar

¼ teaspoon baking soda

1 cup almond milk

1 cup (2 sticks) unsalted butter, melted

2 large eggs, yolks and whites separated

1 teaspoon gluten-free vanilla extract

FOR THE GLAZE

1½ cups powdered sugar

5 tablespoons almond milk, plus more as needed

My grandmother makes her donuts baked and glazed, the way she remembers them. Fluffy rings of dough baked to golden perfection and coated in smooth icing brought back fond childhood memories, and she passed them on in this recipe.

1. **To make the donuts:** Preheat the oven to 350°F. Spray a donut pan with gluten-free cooking spray (see pro tip).

2. In a large bowl, combine the flour blend, sugar, flaxseed meal, baking powder, xanthan gum, cream of tartar, and baking soda. Add the almond milk, butter, egg yolks, and vanilla and mix well.

3. In a separate bowl, beat the egg whites with a hand mixer on medium speed for about 1 minute, until frothy. Add to the flour mixture and stir until combined.

4. Fill each donut well about halfway full. Bake for 8 to 10 minutes, or until the edges are golden brown and a toothpick inserted into the center of a donut comes out clean.

CONTINUED

5. **To make the glaze:** In a small bowl, combine the powdered sugar and almond milk. Use a hand mixer on low speed to mix until completely smooth, adding 1 tablespoon of almond milk to thin, if needed.

6. Remove the donuts from the oven and cool for 5 minutes in the pan before transferring to a wire rack to cool completely. Drizzle with the icing and serve.

7. Store leftovers in an airtight container at room temperature for up to 1 week.

PRO TIP: If you don't have a donut pan, pour the batter into the cups of a muffin tin, filling the cups two-thirds full so they can fluff up during baking. Once cooked, spread the glaze over the tops for delicious glazed muffins.

OOEY GOOEY CINNAMON ROLLS

{ MAKES 12 ROLLS }

PREP TIME: 20 minutes,
plus 1 hour to proof

COOK TIME: 15 minutes

FOR THE CINNAMON ROLLS

1¾ cups All-Purpose Flour Blend
(page 171)

½ teaspoon salt

½ teaspoon xanthan gum

1 (0.75-ounce) package
instant yeast

½ cup milk

¼ cup honey

2 tablespoons unsalted
butter, softened

1 large egg, room temperature

½ teaspoon apple cider vinegar

FOR THE FILLING AND ICING

½ cup sugar

2 tablespoons ground cinnamon

⅓ cup (5⅓ tablespoons) unsalted
butter, melted

1 cup Quick and Easy Icing
(page 168)

If you get as jealous as I did every time you walk by a Cinnabon after giving up gluten and want these delicious morsels back in your life, now's your chance. Enjoy these sweet treats again, only gluten-free.

1. **To make the cinnamon rolls:** Preheat the oven to 350°F and set a rack in the center position. Spray a pie pan with gluten-free cooking spray.

2. In the bowl of a stand mixer fitted with a dough hook or a large bowl with a hand mixer, combine the flour blend, salt, and xanthan gum. Use a finger to poke a small hole in the middle of the flour mixture, then pour the yeast into the hole.

3. Warm the milk to around 115°F in the microwave, using a thermometer to check the temperature (it usually takes 30 to 45 seconds, depending on the microwave).

4. Pour the warm milk over the yeast, then add the honey, butter, egg, and vinegar. Mix until fully combined, about 2 minutes.

5. Cover the bowl with a clean kitchen towel and allow the rolls to proof in a warm place for 1 hour, or until doubled in size.

CONTINUED

6. **To make the filling and icing:** In a small bowl, combine the sugar, cinnamon, and melted butter. Mix well.

7. Spray a large piece of parchment paper with gluten-free cooking spray and transfer the dough onto it. Roll out the dough into a 10-by-16-inch rectangle, about ¼ inch thick.

8. Using the back of a spoon, spread a thin, even layer of filling over the dough.

9. Lifting the end of the parchment paper upward, guide one of the long ends of the dough over itself to form the beginnings of a roll. Continue to lift the parchment paper away from the counter, allowing the dough to roll onto itself until it is one large log.

10. Coat a sharp knife in gluten-free cooking spray and cut the log into 12 equal-size rolls. Arrange the rolls spiral-side up in the bottom of the pie pan.

11. Bake for 16 to 18 minutes, until the edges of the rolls start to turn golden and are slightly firm to the touch, with soft, moist centers.

12. Remove from the oven and cool for 5 to 10 minutes before drizzling with icing. Serve warm.

13. Store leftovers in an airtight container in the refrigerator for up to 3 days.

PRO TIP: When slicing the rolls, cut in one swift motion. Don't use a sawing motion or the swirls may come unraveled.

OVERNIGHT FRENCH TOAST CASSEROLE

{ SERVES 8 }

VT

PREP TIME: 15 minutes, plus 8 hours to chill

COOK TIME: 45 minutes

1 loaf gluten-free bread, cubed

⅓ cup chopped pecans or walnuts

7 large eggs

2 cups milk or full-fat coconut milk

¼ cup honey or maple syrup

1½ tablespoons gluten-free vanilla extract

2½ teaspoons ground cinnamon, divided

½ teaspoon ground nutmeg (optional)

5 tablespoons cold unsalted butter, sliced

½ cup packed light brown sugar

Powdered sugar, for serving (optional)

Start your morning off right with a French toast–inspired casserole dish you prepare the night before. In the morning, all you need to do is sprinkle the cinnamon-sugar crumble on top and bake. Soft and tender on the bottom, crisp and sweet on the top, this recipe is gooey, comforting cinnamon perfection.

1. Spray a 9-by-13-inch baking dish with gluten-free cooking spray. Place the bread cubes in the bottom of the dish and sprinkle with the nuts.

2. In a medium bowl, combine the eggs, milk, honey, vanilla, 1½ teaspoons of cinnamon, and the nutmeg (if using). Mix well. Pour the egg mixture over the bread and stir to coat. Cover with aluminum foil and refrigerate overnight.

3. Preheat the oven to 375°F and remove the dish from the refrigerator.

4. In a small bowl, combine the remaining 1 teaspoon of cinnamon, cold butter slices, and brown sugar. Use a fork to incorporate the ingredients until well combined and crumbly. Sprinkle the mixture over top of the casserole and place the foil back on the dish.

CONTINUED

5. Bake, covered, for 25 minutes, then uncover and continue baking for an additional 20 minutes, until golden brown and heated through.

6. Cool for at least 5 minutes before cutting into squares. Dust with powdered sugar (if using), and serve warm.

7. Store leftovers in an airtight container in the refrigerator for up to 3 days.

PRO TIP: Just like a marinade, the longer this dish sits in the refrigerator, the more the bread will soak up that delicious sauce. Refrigerating overnight is best, but if you don't have that much time, give it at least an hour or two.

WARM CHEESY GRITS
{ SERVES 4 TO 6 }

NF

PREP TIME: 5 minutes

COOK TIME: Per package
directions

2¼ cups milk

1¾ cups gluten-free low-sodium
chicken broth

½ teaspoon salt, plus more
for serving

¼ teaspoon freshly ground black
pepper, plus more for serving

1 cup quick or regular grits (not
instant grits)

1 cup shredded cheddar cheese

4 tablespoons unsalted
butter, sliced

If you're not familiar, grits are corn that has
been ground into a meal. Grits are traditionally
boiled with milk and butter. You can serve this
traditional Southern breakfast staple savory
or sweet. This recipe keeps it hearty with a
generous helping of cheese.

1. In a large saucepan over medium heat,
   combine the milk, broth, salt, and pepper and
   bring to a simmer. Add the grits and mix well.

2. Reduce the heat to low, cover, and cook
   per package directions. Uncover and stir
   continuously for 1 minute. Add the cheese and
   continue stirring for an additional 1 minute,
   then remove from the heat.

3. Divide the grits equally among serving bowls,
   top with a slice of butter, and season with salt
   and pepper.

4. Store leftovers in an airtight container in the
   refrigerator for up to 4 days.

PRO TIP: If you like your grits thicker, reduce the broth by
¼ cup. If you prefer them a bit runnier, add an additional ¼
cup of broth.

VEGETABLE DUTCH BABY

{ SERVES 6 }

PREP TIME: 10 minutes

COOK TIME: 15 minutes

1½ cups tapioca flour

1 cup shredded Swiss cheese

¾ cup heavy (whipping) cream

3 large eggs

1 teaspoon xanthan gum

4 tablespoons (½ stick)
salted butter

1 cup finely chopped fresh
vegetables of choice (such
as asparagus, bell peppers,
mushrooms, onion, or broccoli)

4 tablespoons freshly grated
Parmesan cheese, divided

Pinch freshly ground black pepper

PRO TIP: You might not think the
Dutch baby is done in the middle
when you take it out of the oven,
but as soon as the edges become
golden brown, it's done. The center
will look moist and doughy, but
it will set after a few minutes of
cooling. Be sure not to overcook.

Is it a pancake or a pie? Neither—and both. A
Dutch baby is a combination of pancake, doughy
biscuit, and simple pie, often topped with fruit
and sprinkled in powdered sugar. I prefer this
comfort favorite savory, however, which is why
I've loaded it with veggies and cheese. Dutch
babies are typically served in slices like a pie
during the first half of the day, but you can eat
yours however and whenever you like (I won't
tell the Dutch).

1. Preheat the oven to 425°F.

2. In a large bowl, whisk together the tapioca
    flour, Swiss cheese, cream, eggs, and
    xanthan gum.

3. In a large oven-safe skillet, melt the butter
    over medium heat. Remove from the heat and
    carefully pour in the batter.

4. Sprinkle the chopped vegetables and
    2 tablespoons of Parmesan cheese on top. Bake
    for 12 to 15 minutes, or until golden brown and
    bubbly around the edges.

5. Sprinkle the remaining 2 tablespoons of
    Parmesan cheese and pepper on top and
    serve warm.

QUICK EGG MUFFINS

{ MAKES 12 MUFFINS }

NF 30

PREP TIME: 10 minutes

COOK TIME: 20 minutes

5 large eggs

1½ tablespoons milk

¼ teaspoon freshly ground black pepper

¼ teaspoon garlic salt

2 ounces goat cheese, crumbled

Handful baby spinach, chopped

Handful grape tomatoes, halved

¼ small sweet onion, chopped

1 precooked breakfast sausage link, thinly sliced

¾ teaspoon paprika, for garnish

PRO TIP: Use any meat or veggies you have on hand. Substitute bacon or ham for the sausage, and try broccoli, kale, sweet potato, or bell pepper for the vegetables.

These protein-packed egg muffins combine the flavor punch of savory breakfast sausage, tangy goat cheese, juicy tomatoes, and a few sweet onion slices. They are a portable, delicious way to fuel your morning.

1. Preheat the oven to 375°F. Spray a 12-cup muffin tin with gluten-free cooking spray.

2. In a large bowl, whisk together the eggs, milk, pepper, and garlic salt.

3. Sprinkle equal parts goat cheese, spinach, tomato, onion, and sausage into each of the 12 muffin cups.

4. Divide the egg mixture equally among the muffin cups (it should almost reach the top), and stir each cup. Sprinkle each cup with a pinch of paprika.

5. Bake for 20 to 25 minutes, or until the eggs are fully cooked and golden brown around the edges.

6. Cool for 1 to 2 minutes. Run a knife around the edge of each egg muffin and remove from the pan. Serve immediately.

7. Store leftovers in an airtight container in the refrigerator for up to 1 week or in the freezer for up to 4 months.

HAM AND CHEESE QUICHE

{ SERVES 8 }

NF

PREP TIME: 10 minutes

COOK TIME: 40 minutes

1 (9-inch) frozen
gluten-free piecrust

1 tablespoon unsalted butter

½ cup diced sweet onion

1½ cups diced ham

1½ cups shredded cheddar cheese

1¼ cups milk

4 large eggs

½ teaspoon garlic powder

2 thinly sliced scallions, for serving

PRO TIP: To make this recipe
dairy-free, substitute olive oil
for the butter and use dairy-free
shredded cheese.

If you're the type of person who likes to eat breakfast for every meal, this quiche is for you. With the combination of rich cheese, sweet onions, and a generous helping of meat baked inside a buttery crust, you won't even notice that the dish is gluten-free. Enjoy this savory breakfast treat any hour of the day.

1. Preheat the oven to 375°F. Place the frozen piecrust onto a large rimmed baking sheet.

2. In a medium skillet, melt the butter over medium heat. Add the onion and cook for 3 to 4 minutes, stirring occasionally, until fragrant and translucent. Remove from the heat.

3. In a large bowl, combine the ham, cheese, milk, eggs, and garlic powder and stir. Add the onions and mix thoroughly.

4. Pour the mixture into the piecrust and bake for 33 to 37 minutes, until the top is golden brown and the center is only slightly wobbly.

5. Cool for 5 minutes before cutting into slices. Sprinkle each slice with scallions and serve.

6. Store leftovers in an airtight container in the refrigerator for up to 3 days.

BREAKFAST ENCHILADAS

{ SERVES 8 }

NF

PREP TIME: 15 minutes

COOK TIME: 45 minutes

3 tablespoons unsalted butter, softened, divided

9 large eggs

½ pound gluten-free ground breakfast sausage

3 bacon slices

1 cup buttermilk

1 tablespoon All-Purpose Flour Blend (page 171)

½ teaspoon garlic powder

1 cup shredded cheddar cheese, divided

8 gluten-free corn tortillas

¼ cup grape tomatoes, halved

2 tablespoons chopped scallions

Who says enchiladas are strictly for dinner? Breakfast sausage and fluffy eggs rolled into tortillas and drizzled with the most decadent cheese sauce sounds like *exactly* the way I want to start my morning. Even better, the whole dish is sprinkled with bacon, tomatoes, and scallions. Get ready to ramp up your breakfast routine.

1. Preheat the oven to 375°F.

2. In a large skillet, melt 1 tablespoon of butter over low heat, turning to coat the pan. Beat the eggs, pour them in the pan, and cook for about 4 minutes, stirring regularly to scramble, until just cooked (they should still be slightly runny). Transfer to a large bowl.

3. Increase the heat to medium and place the sausage and bacon in the skillet. Cook for 15 minutes, turning occasionally, until both meats are deep golden and cooked through. Transfer the bacon to a plate lined with paper towels. Drain the sausage and add it to the eggs, mixing well.

CONTINUED ᕦ

4. In a medium saucepan over medium heat, combine the buttermilk, flour blend, and remaining 2 tablespoons of butter. Bring to a simmer. Add the garlic powder and continue to simmer for 3 to 5 minutes, stirring occasionally, until the sauce starts to thicken. Add ¾ cup shredded cheese and stir until smooth, 2 to 3 minutes. Remove from the heat.

5. Scoop about one-eighth of the egg mixture into a tortilla and roll it up like a cigar, then place it in a large baking dish, seam-side down. Repeat with the remaining tortillas and egg mixture, placing the rolls next to each other, until the dish is full. Smother the entire dish with the cheese sauce, and sprinkle the remaining ¼ cup shredded cheese on top.

6. Bake for 20 to 25 minutes, or until the tortillas are golden brown around the edges.

7. Remove from the oven and top with the tomatoes and scallions, then crumble the bacon over the top. Serve hot.

8. Store leftovers in an airtight container in the refrigerator for up to 3 days.

PRO TIP: This recipe is a great way to use up leftover meat from last night's dinner. You can put pretty much anything in these enchiladas.

SOUTHERN SKILLET FRITTATA

{ SERVES 8 }

DF NF

PREP TIME: 10 minutes

COOK TIME: 30 minutes

8 bacon slices

3 tablespoons cooking oil, such as olive, coconut, or canola

1 medium sweet potato, cut into ¾-inch cubes

1 cup chopped kale or spinach

½ cup diced onion

½ teaspoon minced garlic

1 teaspoon dried thyme or 3 teaspoons chopped fresh thyme

½ teaspoon garlic powder

8 fresh sage leaves, chopped, or ½ teaspoon dried sage

¼ teaspoon paprika

Salt

Freshly ground black pepper

8 large eggs

2 tablespoons water

This recipe is a great choice when you host a brunch. It is easy to make, creates the most enticingly fragrant aromas, and is visually stunning—hard for any guest to resist. You will have friends and family lined up to get a slice of this savory treat.

1. Preheat the oven to 375°F.

2. On a rimmed baking sheet, lay out the bacon slices. Bake for 15 to 20 minutes, or until the outer edges are dark brown and the center of each slice is golden brown with a ribbon-like ripple shape. Remove from the heat and transfer to a plate lined with paper towels. Let the bacon cool, then chop into 1-inch pieces.

3. In an oven-safe skillet, warm the oil over medium heat, moving the pan to coat the bottom and sides of the skillet. Add the sweet potato and cook for about 10 minutes, stirring occasionally, until fork-tender.

4. Add the bacon, kale, onion, garlic, thyme, garlic powder, sage, paprika, and salt and pepper to taste. Cook for about 5 minutes, until the kale has wilted.

CONTINUED 🍃

5.   Beat the eggs with the water. Reduce the heat to low and add the eggs, stirring until thoroughly mixed. Cook, undisturbed, for 4 to 5 minutes, or until the egg just starts to set.

6.   Transfer to the oven and bake for an additional 10 to 12 minutes, or until the edges are golden brown and pulling away from the skillet.

7.   Cool for 5 minutes before slicing and serving.

8.   Store leftovers in an airtight container in the refrigerator for up to 3 days.

PRO TIP: To make this a visual masterpiece, sprinkle the top of the frittata with a few extra pieces of bacon, onion, paprika, or sage leaves before slipping it into the oven. Once the frittata is out of the oven, top with a few fresh sprigs of thyme.

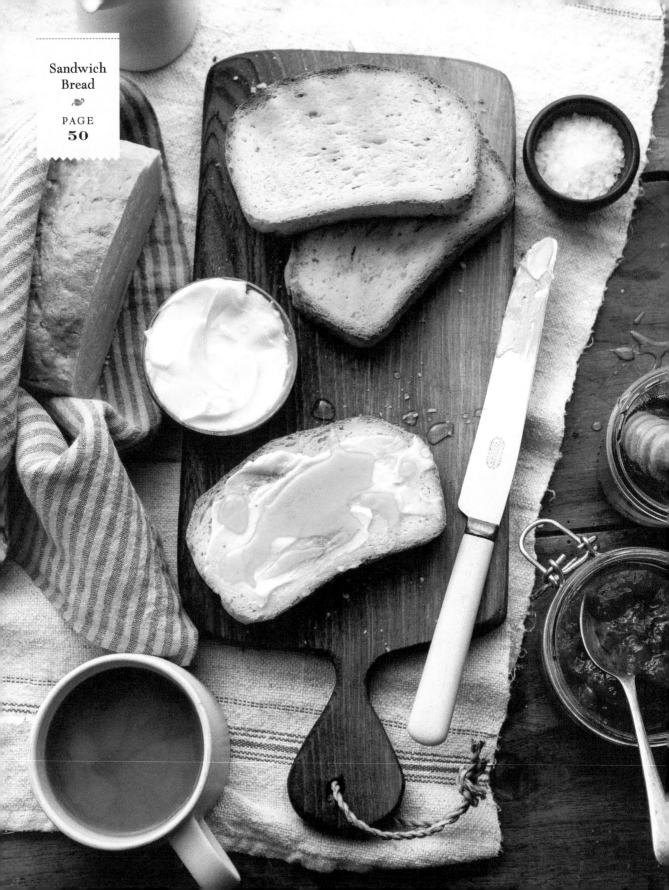

Sandwich
Bread

PAGE
50

{ 03 }
BREADS AND CRACKERS

CRUNCHY GRAHAM CRACKERS

{ MAKES 24 GRAHAM CRACKERS }

DF   VT

PREP TIME: 10 minutes,
plus 30 minutes to chill

COOK TIME: 15 minutes

2¼ cups almond flour

½ cup packed light brown sugar

1 teaspoon baking powder

1 teaspoon ground cinnamon

½ teaspoon fine sea salt

1 large egg

2 tablespoons honey

2 tablespoons coconut oil

PRO TIP: Use a pizza cutter
to make quick, straight lines in
the dough.

Feel like you're missing out during s'mores
season? I felt the same way until I discovered how
deliciously wonderful homemade gluten-free
graham crackers can be.

1. In a large bowl, combine the almond flour,
    brown sugar, baking powder, cinnamon, and
    salt. Mix well.

2. Add the egg, honey, and oil and stir until well
    combined. Place the bowl in the refrigerator
    for 30 minutes to chill.

3. Preheat the oven to 325°F. Line a large rimless
    baking sheet with parchment paper.

4. Place the dough on the paper, and place an
    equal-size sheet of parchment paper over
    the top of the dough. Use a rolling pin to roll
    the dough into an 11-by-14-inch rectangle,
    ¼ to ⅛ inch thick. Remove the top sheet of
    parchment paper and cut the dough into
    24 equal-size rectangles.

5. Bake for 12 to 14 minutes, or until the edges
    turn golden but the centers are still soft.
    Remove from the oven and cool for 5 minutes
    on the baking sheet before transferring to a
    wire rack to cool completely.

CRISPY CHEESE CRACKERS

{ MAKES 8 CRACKERS }

NF VT

PREP TIME: 15 minutes, plus 10 minutes to chill

COOK TIME: 15 minutes

1 cup All-Purpose Flour Blend (page 171)

1 cup shredded sharp cheddar cheese

4½ tablespoons unsalted butter, softened

1 tablespoon coarse sea salt

PRO TIP: Use a pizza cutter to make quick, straight lines in the dough before and after you bake the crackers.

Made from just four simple ingredients, these cheesy, buttery crackers have the perfect crunch in every bite. The sprinkling of coarse salt right before baking gives these crackers a flake-in-your-mouth, addictive goodness.

1. In a food processor, combine the flour blend, cheese, and butter. Process for 1 to 2 minutes, until a dough forms.

2. Remove the dough from the food processor and wrap in plastic wrap. Refrigerate for 10 minutes to chill.

3. Preheat the oven to 350°F. Spray a rimless baking sheet and a rolling pin with gluten-free cooking spray.

4. Working quickly so as not to warm the chilled dough, roll out the dough onto the baking sheet into a 4-by-8-inch rectangle, about ¼ inch thick. Cut the dough into 8 (1-inch) squares. Sprinkle generously with salt.

5. Bake for 13 to 15 minutes, until the edges of the dough start to turn a darker golden color.

6. Remove from the oven and cool in the pan for 1 to 2 minutes before slicing along the cut marks. Transfer to a wire rack to cool completely.

THIN PIZZA CRUST

{ MAKES 2 (10-INCH) PIZZA CRUSTS }

PREP TIME: 20 minutes

COOK TIME: 10 minutes

1¾ cups plus 2 tablespoons
All-Purpose Flour Blend (page 171)

½ teaspoon salt

½ teaspoon xanthan gum

1 (0.75-ounce) package
instant yeast

½ cup plus 2 tablespoons milk

2 tablespoons unsalted
butter, softened

1 large egg, room temperature

2 tablespoons honey

½ teaspoon apple cider vinegar

This thin pizza crust is so simple and quick, you'll be asking yourself why you haven't been making your own crust all this time.

In about 30 minutes, this recipe provides the base for a made-from-scratch gluten-free pizza with all your favorite toppings—right at home.

1. Preheat the oven to 450°F.

2. In the bowl of a stand mixer fitted with a dough hook or a large bowl with a hand mixer, combine the flour blend, salt, and xanthan gum. Use your finger to poke a small hole in the middle of the flour mixture, then pour the yeast into the hole.

3. Warm the milk to around 115°F in the microwave, checking the temperature with a thermometer (it usually takes between 30 and 45 seconds, depending on the microwave). Pour the warm milk over the yeast.

4. Add the butter, egg, honey, and vinegar, and mix until fully combined, about 2 minutes.

5. Spray a large baking sheet and your hands with gluten-free cooking spray.

6. Place half the dough on one half of the baking sheet, and flatten it into a large disk, approximately 10 inches across and ¼ inch thick. Repeat with the other half of the dough on the other half of the baking sheet or another baking sheet.

7. Parbake the pizza crust on the middle rack for 6 to 7 minutes, until the edges begin to harden but the center still looks uncooked. Remove from the oven and add the toppings to cook (see Pepperoni Pizza, page 114), or let cool completely before wrapping in plastic wrap.

8. Store parbaked dough in the refrigerator for up to 24 hours or in the freezer for up to 2 weeks.

PRO TIP: This is a great make-ahead recipe. Feel free to make multiples of this crust for a party. I usually make 4 to 6 pizza crusts (that's 2 to 3 full batches) at one time, even if I'm not feeding a group—I just freeze any crusts I won't be using right away.

SOFT FLOUR TORTILLAS

{ MAKES 10 (8-INCH) TORTILLAS }

PREP TIME: 20 minutes,
plus 20 minutes to chill

COOK TIME: 10 minutes

1 cup milk

2½ cups tapioca flour, plus more
for sprinkling

⅛ teaspoon salt

3 tablespoons olive oil

1 room temperature egg, beaten

8 ounces mozzarella
cheese, shredded

2 ounces Parmesan cheese, grated

Unlike many store-bought gluten-free tortillas, these don't crumble into a million pieces or become soggy seconds after you fill them. Stuff these thick tortillas with your favorite burrito ingredients, use them as wraps with your favorite fixings, or cut a slit in the top and create a pita pocket!

1. In a medium saucepan, warm the milk over medium heat until simmering. Remove from the heat, add the tapioca flour and salt, and mix thoroughly.

2. Add the oil and return to the heat, mixing until it becomes slightly chunky. Remove from the heat and let cool for 15 minutes.

3. Transfer the cooled mixture to a food processor. Pulse until the dough is smooth. Add the egg and pulse for an additional 1 to 2 minutes, until smooth. Add the mozzarella and Parmesan cheese and pulse for an additional 1 to 2 minutes, until smooth.

4. Wet your hands and divide the dough into two halves. Wrap the dough in plastic wrap and place in the freezer for 20 to 25 minutes to chill.

5. Sprinkle a clean, flat surface with tapioca flour. Remove one of the dough halves from the freezer and divide it into 5 sections on the floured surface. Use a rolling pin to roll each into a disk approximately 8 inches across. Dust the disks with tapioca flour as needed to prevent sticking.

6. Heat a large nonstick skillet over medium heat. Place a tortilla in the pan and cook for 60 to 90 seconds on both sides, until lightly browned. The tortilla should lift easily from the skillet when done. (Pressing down with a spatula may speed the cooking process.) Repeat with the remaining 4 disks of dough.

7. Remove the other half of the dough from the freezer and repeat steps 5 and 6.

8. Store leftovers in an airtight container in the refrigerator for up to 5 days.

PRO TIP: Make these tortillas in bulk and freeze them for later—they stay amazing each and every time. For extended storing, wrap each tortilla tightly in aluminum foil, slide them into a freezer-safe plastic bag, and press out all the extra air. They'll stay good for up to 2 months in the freezer.

BASIC FLATBREAD
{ SERVES 4 }

PREP TIME: 15 minutes

COOK TIME: 10 minutes

1¾ cups All-Purpose Flour Blend (page 171)

½ teaspoon salt

½ teaspoon xanthan gum

1 (0.75-ounce) package instant yeast

½ cup milk

2 tablespoons unsalted butter, softened

1 large egg, room temperature

1 tablespoon honey

½ teaspoon apple cider vinegar

This recipe produces a quick, easy, partly baked flatbread you can finish however (and whenever) you like (see pro tip). Toss your favorite vegetables or cheeses on top and stick the flatbread back into the oven. *Voilà!* So easy, and it will be a hit everywhere you serve it.

1. Preheat the oven to 450°F and set a rack in the center position.

2. In the bowl of a stand mixer fitted with a dough hook or a large bowl with a hand mixer, combine the flour blend, salt, and xanthan gum. Use your finger to poke a small hole in the middle of the flour mixture, then pour the yeast into the hole.

3. Warm the milk to around 115°F in the microwave, using a thermometer to check the temperature (it usually takes between 30 and 45 seconds, depending on the microwave). Pour the warm milk over the yeast.

4. Add the butter, egg, honey, and vinegar and mix until fully combined, about 2 minutes.

5. Spray a large baking sheet and your hands with gluten-free cooking spray. Place the dough on the baking sheet and flatten it into an 8-by-16-inch rectangle, about ¼ inch thick.

6. Parbake the flatbread for 6 minutes, until the edges look crisp but the center is still doughy. Remove from the heat and add the toppings, then return to the oven and bake for 4 to 5 additional minutes, until the toppings are hot. If saving for later, wrap tightly with plastic wrap, place in a freezer-safe bag, and refrigerate for up to 48 hours.

PRO TIP: For a delicious cheesy pesto flatbread, sprinkle 1 cup of chopped spinach on top of the dough, along with 2 tablespoons of gluten-free pesto and 2 cups of shredded mozzarella cheese. Place the flatbread back into the preheated 450°F oven for 4 to 5 minutes, until the cheese has melted and turned golden brown around the edges.

SANDWICH BREAD

{ MAKES 1 (5-BY-9-INCH) LOAF }

PREP TIME: 20 minutes,
plus 1 hour to proof

COOK TIME: 45 minutes

¾ cup water

1 (0.75-ounce) package
instant yeast

3 large egg whites

¼ cup olive oil

1½ tablespoons apple cider vinegar

3 cups All-Purpose Flour Blend
(page 171)

¼ cup packed light brown sugar

2¼ teaspoons xanthan gum

½ teaspoon baking powder

How many times have you tried a piece of
gluten-free bread only to be disappointed? Say
goodbye to brittle, crumbly, tasteless bread and
hello to sandwich heaven!

1. Spray a 5-by-9-inch glass loaf pan with
    gluten-free cooking spray. (This recipe tends to
    stick to the sides of metal pans.)

2. In a large microwave-safe bowl, micro-
    wave the water to around 115°F, using a
    thermometer to check the temperature (it
    usually takes between 30 and 45 seconds).
    Place the yeast in the warm water and
    stir gently.

3. Place the egg whites in the bowl of a stand
    mixer fitted with the whisk attachment or in
    a large bowl. Whisk or beat on medium-high
    speed until stiff peaks form, 5 to 7 minutes.

4. Reduce the mixer speed to medium. Add
    the oil and vinegar, then slowly pour in the
    yeast mixture. Add the flour blend, brown
    sugar, xanthan gum, and baking powder and
    continue mixing until a smooth dough forms,
    1 to 3 minutes.

5. Place the dough in the loaf pan. Cover with a
    clean kitchen towel and allow the dough to rise
    in a warm place for 1 hour, or until doubled
    in size.

6. During the last 10 minutes of proofing, preheat the oven to 350°F and set a rack in the center position.

7. Bake for 45 minutes, until the edges are golden brown and the top has hardened into a golden crust. Cool for 2 to 3 minutes in the pan before transferring to a wire rack to cool completely. Slice and serve.

Simple Egg Yolk Mayonnaise

Turn the leftover egg yolks from this recipe into homemade mayo!

2 large egg yolks

1 tablespoon Dijon mustard

1½ cups olive oil, divided

2 tablespoons vinegar (white wine vinegar recommended)

2 teaspoons freshly squeezed lemon juice

½ teaspoon salt

⅛ teaspoon sugar

1. In a medium mixing bowl, whisk the egg yolks and mustard. Over the course of 4 to 5 minutes, add half the oil, whisking all the while.

2. Whisk in the vinegar and slowly add in the rest of the oil, whisking continuously. Add the lemon juice, salt, and sugar and whisk for an additional 30 seconds.

SAVORY POTATO ROLLS

{ MAKES 24 ROLLS }

PREP TIME: 10 minutes

COOK TIME: 10 minutes

1 cup All-Purpose Flour Blend
(page 171)

1 cup plain mashed potatoes or
instant potatoes

2 large eggs, room temperature

¼ cup nutritional yeast flakes

¾ teaspoon salt

PRO TIP: You can also make these
rolls in a regular muffin tin. Place
clementine-size portions of dough
into each muffin cup and increase
the baking time to 12 to 16 minutes.
If you want the tops of the rolls
to be nice and smooth, spray the
back of a spatula or spoon with
gluten-free cooking spray and
gently glide it along the top of
each roll before baking.

Whenever we had dinner at Grandma's
house, she always served up a fresh basket of
ridiculously moist potato rolls that no one could
pass up. This recipe for doughy potato rolls
brings back this classic in miniature form—the
perfect addition to your dinner table. This recipe
uses nutritional yeast. It's a crumbly dairy-free
ingredient that still tastes deliciously cheesy and
is also a complete protein, so it's a great stand-in
for Parmesan cheese (but you can use powdered
Parmesan, too).

1. Preheat the oven to 425°F. Spray a 24-cup mini
   muffin tin with gluten-free cooking spray.

2. In a large bowl, mix together the flour blend,
   potatoes, eggs, nutritional yeast, and salt until
   a dough forms.

3. Place a ping pong ball–size portion of dough
   into each muffin cup.

4. Bake for 8 to 12 minutes, or until the tops start
   to turn golden brown. Cool for 1 to 2 minutes
   in the pan before transferring to a wire rack to
   cool completely.

5. Store leftovers in an airtight container at room
   temperature for up to 3 days.

ZUCCHINI BREAD

{ MAKES 1 (5-BY-9-INCH) LOAF }

PREP TIME: 15 minutes

COOK TIME: 50 minutes

All-Purpose Flour Blend
(page 171), for dusting

2¾ cups zucchini
(2 or 3 medium zucchini)

½ large sweet onion

2 large eggs

¼ cup olive oil

¼ cup heavy (whipping) cream

¾ cup shredded Parmesan cheese

1½ cups Biscuit Mix (page 172)

PRO TIP: To squeeze the extra
liquid from the zucchini-onion
mixture, transfer it onto the center
of a clean kitchen towel. Standing
over the sink, gather the sides
of the towel and twist to seal,
tightening it into a ball shape until
the liquids begin to drain. Squeeze
until no more liquids come from
the mixture.

Zucchini bread is one of the tastiest and most fun
breads to make and eat. Kids love to help because
it's a blast to squish the zucchini between little
fingers, and everyone will savor the amazing
smell coming from the oven.

1. Preheat the oven to 350°F. Spray a 5-by-9-inch
    loaf pan with gluten-free cooking spray and
    dust with the flour blend.

2. Place the zucchini and onion in a food pro-
    cessor and process until finely diced, then
    squeeze out the extra moisture (see pro tip).

3. In a large bowl, combine the eggs, oil, and
    cream and mix until well blended.

4. Add the squeezed zucchini-onion mixture,
    cheese, and biscuit mix. Stir until well blended.
    Pour the batter into the loaf pan.

5. Bake for 50 to 60 minutes, or until the edges
    are golden brown and a toothpick inserted into
    the center of the loaf comes out clean.

6. Cool in the pan for 5 minutes before
    transferring to a wire rack. Cool for an
    additional 10 to 15 minutes before slicing
    and serving.

7. Store leftovers in an airtight container at room
    temperature for up to 5 days.

EASY PAN ROLLS

{ MAKES 9 ROLLS }

NF VT

PREP TIME: 20 minutes,
plus 1 hour to proof

COOK TIME: 15 minutes

1¾ cups All-Purpose Flour Blend
(page 171)

½ teaspoon salt

½ teaspoon xanthan gum

1 (0.75-ounce) package
instant yeast

½ cup plus 2 tablespoons milk

2 tablespoons unsalted butter,
softened, plus 2 tablespoons
melted butter for brushing

1 large egg, room temperature

¼ cup honey

½ teaspoon apple cider vinegar

Growing up, I loved creating dishes in the
kitchen. When it came to baking, however,
I lacked expertise and confidence. I always felt
completely comfortable with drop biscuits,
though, because there was no kneading or rolling
involved. Today I am still much more comfortable
cooking than baking, but these rolls will increase
your baking self-confidence once and for all.
These fluffy, buttery dinner rolls couldn't be any
more delicious or easier to make.

1. In the bowl of a stand mixer fitted with a
    dough hook or a large bowl with a hand mixer,
    combine the flour blend, salt, and xanthan
    gum. Use your finger to poke a small hole in
    the middle of the flour mixture, then pour the
    yeast into the hole.

2. Warm the milk to around 115°F in the
    microwave, using a thermometer to check the
    temperature (it usually takes between 30 and
    45 seconds, depending on the microwave).
    Pour the warm milk over the yeast.

3. Add the 2 tablespoons of softened butter,
    egg, honey, and vinegar and mix until fully
    combined, about 2 minutes.

4. Spray a 9-inch square baking dish with
    gluten-free cooking spray.

5. Spray an ice cream scoop with gluten-free cooking spray. Scoop 9 equal-size balls of dough into the dish.

6. Cover the pan with a clean kitchen towel and allow the rolls to proof in a warm place for 1 hour, or until doubled in size.

7. During the last 10 minutes of proofing, preheat the oven to 400°F and set a rack in the center position. Bake the rolls for 11 to 13 minutes, until the edges turn a warm golden brown.

8. Cool in the pan for 2 to 3 minutes. Just before serving, brush the tops of the rolls with the melted butter.

9. Store leftovers in an airtight container at room temperature for up to 5 days.

PRO TIP: For smooth, shiny rolls, place cool water on a spatula and run it over the top of each roll before baking.

MINI BUTTERMILK BISCUITS

{ MAKES 24 BISCUITS }

PREP TIME: 10 minutes

COOK TIME: 10 minutes

2 cups Biscuit Mix (page 172)

1 tablespoon baking powder

1 teaspoon xanthan gum

6 tablespoons cold unsalted butter, cubed

1 cup buttermilk

Nothing says comfort like buttery biscuits. These fluffy, moist miniature biscuits are soft and tender bite after bite, and they'll please everyone at the dinner table. They partner perfectly with your favorite soup or Easy Beef Stew (page 90), as a side next to your hot breakfast, or to the side of a meaty dish such as Fried Chicken and Waffles (page 102) or Pork Chops and Gravy (page 131).

1. Preheat the oven to 425°F. Spray a 24-cup mini muffin tin with gluten-free cooking spray.

2. In a large bowl, combine the biscuit mix, baking powder, and xanthan gum. Add the butter and use your hands to work the mixture together until it resembles small pebbles. Add the buttermilk and stir until a dough is formed.

3. Using your hands, roll a piece of dough until it is the size of a large gumball. Place one dough ball into each muffin cup.

4. Bake for 8 to 10 minutes, or until the biscuits are golden brown around the edges. Cool for 5 minutes in the pan before transferring to a wire rack to cool completely.

5. Store leftovers in an airtight container at room temperature for up to 3 days.

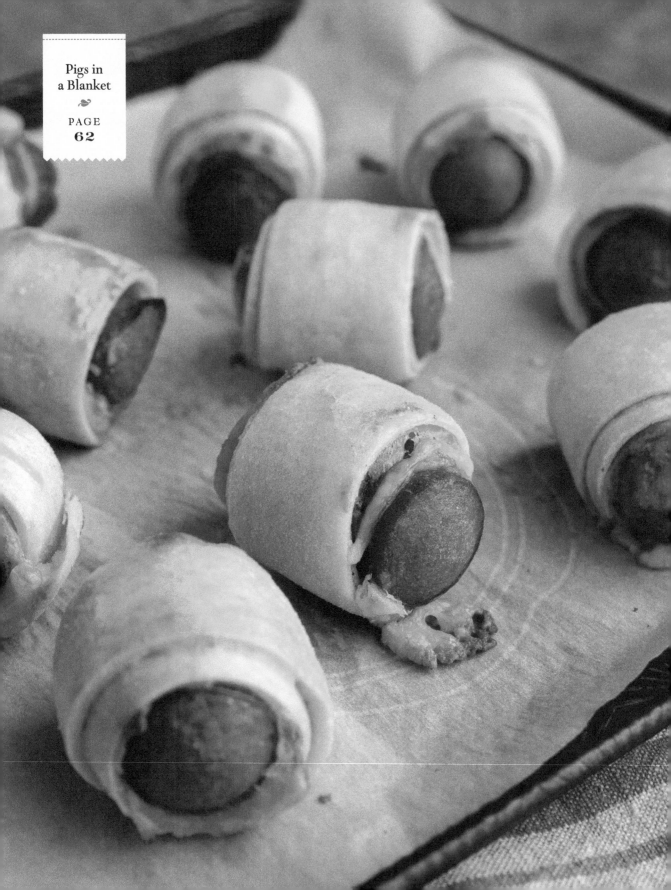

Pigs in
a Blanket

PAGE
62

{ 04 }
SIDES

BREAD AND BUTTER PICKLES

{ SERVES 12 }

PREP TIME: 20 minutes, plus 26 hours to chill

COOK TIME: 10 minutes

3 medium cucumbers, cut into ¼-inch rounds (about 6 cups)

2 teaspoons salt

1 sweet onion, thinly sliced

1 cup white vinegar

½ cup apple cider vinegar

⅔ cup granulated sugar

¼ cup packed light brown sugar

1¾ teaspoons whole mustard seeds

½ teaspoon whole celery seeds

⅛ teaspoon ground turmeric

These fresh, crisp pickles are both sweet and tangy. These jars of pickled cucumbers store well for months in the refrigerator, but be careful—once friends try one, they will be begging for more to bring home.

1. Combine the cucumbers and salt in a large bowl, stirring to coat. Cover and refrigerate for 1 hour.

2. Place the cucumbers in a colander and rinse with cold water. Transfer to a large bowl and add the onion.

3. In a medium saucepan, combine the white vinegar, apple cider vinegar, granulated sugar, brown sugar, mustard seeds, celery seeds, and turmeric. Cook over medium heat until the sugars have dissolved, about 5 minutes.

4. Pour the vinegar mixture over the cucumbers and onion. Let it sit at room temperature for 1 hour. Cover and refrigerate for 24 hours.

5. Store leftovers in an airtight jar in the refrigerator for up to 5 months.

PRO TIP: These pickles make a great gift. Simply wrap the storage jar in burlap and tie a ribbon with a gift tag around its neck. Thoughtful and delicious.

CREAMY COLESLAW

{ SERVES 4 TO 6 }

NF VT 30

PREP TIME: 10 minutes

½ (14-ounce) bag
shredded cabbage

1 apple, peeled, cored, and diced

2 cups chopped kale

6 tablespoons plain yogurt

1 tablespoon Dijon mustard

1 teaspoon coconut sugar or
granulated sugar

1 teaspoon olive oil

1 teaspoon apple cider vinegar

1 teaspoon freshly squeezed
lemon juice

Pinch salt

Need a way to get your kids to eat more greens?
Try mixing up this quick and delicious dish.
Diced vegetables are coated in a yogurt-based
sauce that's been blended with lemon juice and
apple cider vinegar to add a touch of tanginess,
sugar for a pinch of sweet, and Dijon mustard for
a bit of attitude.

1. In a large bowl, mix the cabbage, apple, and
    kale. In a small bowl, mix the yogurt, mustard,
    sugar, oil, vinegar, lemon juice, and salt.

2. Drizzle the sauce over the cabbage mixture
    and toss to combine. Serve immediately or
    allow to chill in the refrigerator until ready
    to enjoy.

3. Store leftovers in an airtight container in the
    refrigerator for up to 3 days.

PRO TIP: Freshen up the leftovers by adding an extra
drop or two of lemon juice and stirring thoroughly.

PIGS IN A BLANKET

{ MAKES 15 }

NF

PREP TIME: 10 minutes, plus 1 hour to proof

COOK TIME: 10 minutes

2½ cups All-Purpose Flour Blend (page 171), plus more for dusting

1 (0.75-ounce) package instant yeast

1½ teaspoons xanthan gum

1¼ teaspoons sugar

¼ teaspoon salt

3 tablespoons olive oil, plus more for drizzling

¾ cup warm water

15 (1-inch) strips cheese (such as sharp cheddar, American, or pepper Jack)

5 gluten-free hot dogs, cut into thirds

PRO TIP: This kid-friendly dish can easily be turned into impressive hors d'oeuvres for adults. Swap out the hot dogs with delicious seasoned pork or chicken sausage links, and up your cheese game with a creamy Gruyère or Gouda.

Pigs in a blanket were one of the foods I missed most when I became gluten-free. There's no missing them anymore, though!

1. In a large bowl, combine the flour blend, yeast, xanthan gum, sugar, and salt.

2. Add the oil and water and mix using a hand mixer on low speed until the dough is well blended. If still sticky, add more flour, 1 tablespoon at a time. Mold the dough into a ball, drizzle all over with oil, cover the bowl with plastic wrap, and let the dough rise in a warm spot for 1 hour.

3. Preheat the oven to 400°F. Line a baking sheet with parchment paper.

4. Divide the dough into 3 equal parts and dust each part well with flour. Roll each part into ⅛- to ¼-inch-thick rectangles. With a knife, cut the rolled-out dough into 5 strips, 2 to 3 inches wide and about 6 inches long.

5. Center one strip of cheese on a strip of dough. Place one hot dog piece over the cheese perpendicular to the dough. Roll up the dough. Place each wrapped hot dog onto the baking sheet, seam-side down, spacing about 1 inch apart.

6. Bake for 10 to 12 minutes, or until the dough starts to turn golden brown along the edges. Enjoy warm.

BAKED SWEET POTATO FRIES

{ SERVES 4 }

DF   NF   V

PREP TIME: 10 minutes

COOK TIME: 40 minutes

2 large sweet potatoes, cut into ½- to 1-inch spears

3 teaspoons olive oil

¼ teaspoon garlic salt

¼ teaspoon garlic powder

Need to get your hands on a salty snack? These from-scratch sweet potato fries will do the trick. Crisp on the outside, tender and warm on the inside, they are baked and not deep-fried, making for a healthier treat.

1. Preheat the oven to 400°F.

2. Lay the sweet potatoes on a large baking pan. Drizzle the oil over the potatoes and use a basting brush to coat them thoroughly.

3. Sprinkle the garlic salt and garlic powder on the potatoes, spreading with the same brush.

4. Bake for 40 minutes, flipping halfway through the baking process. For a crisper fry, turn the oven to broil and cook for a few extra minutes at the end.

5. Store leftovers in an airtight container in the refrigerator for up to 5 days.

PRO TIP: Not a sweet potato fan? Swap them for russet potatoes and shorten the bake time by 2 to 3 minutes.

BLUE CHEESE GREEN BEANS

{ SERVES 4 }

PREP TIME: 5 minutes

COOK TIME: 10 minutes

1 pound fresh green beans, trimmed

¼ cup water

2 teaspoons olive oil

¼ teaspoon freshly ground black pepper

⅓ cup crumbled blue cheese

⅓ cup chopped pecans

If you're a fan of creamy-meets-crunchy savory dishes, you have to try these tender-crisp green beans mixed with toasted nuts and dreamy blue cheese sauce. This 5-ingredient, 15-minute recipe made me fall in love with green beans for the first time. I'm hoping it has the same effect on you.

1. In a large nonstick skillet, bring the green beans and water to a boil over medium heat. Reduce the heat to a simmer, cover, and cook for an additional 2 to 4 minutes. Uncover and continue cooking, stirring occasionally, until the water is evaporated, about 4 minutes. Remove from the heat and add the oil.

2. While still hot, quickly sprinkle the pepper, cheese, and pecans on top and stir to combine, allowing the pecans to toast in the skillet for 2 minutes. Serve immediately.

3. Store leftovers in an airtight container in the refrigerator for up to 48 hours.

PRO TIP: If you want to increase the serving size of this dish for big crowds (or large appetites), double all the ingredients.

CHOPPED MEXICAN STREET CORN SALAD

{ SERVES 4 TO 6 }

PREP TIME: 20 minutes

1 cup white rice

3 (15-ounce) cans sweet corn kernels, drained

1 cup diced tomatoes (or canned diced tomatoes)

1 cup diced bell pepper

¼ cup finely chopped red onion

1 jalapeño, finely chopped (optional)

⅓ cup chopped fresh cilantro

2 tablespoons cooking oil, such as olive, coconut, or canola

1 tablespoon freshly squeezed lime juice

½ teaspoon gluten-free taco seasoning

¼ teaspoon garlic powder

On a hot summer day, what's better than a cool, refreshing salad that also invigorates your palate? Here, sweet corn kernels are tossed with tender rice grains, fresh tomatoes, crisp peppers, fragrant onion pieces, and flecks of fresh cilantro, all topped with a garlicky lime oil drizzle.

1. Cook the rice according to package directions.

2. In a large bowl, combine the rice, corn, tomatoes, bell pepper, onion, jalapeño (if using), and cilantro. Mix well.

3. In a small bowl, combine the oil, lime juice, taco seasoning, and garlic powder. Mix well.

4. Coat the vegetable-rice mixture with the garlic-lime drizzle, mix well, and serve.

5. Store leftovers in an airtight container in the refrigerator for up to 5 days.

PRO TIP: Feel free to garnish this salad with Cotija cheese crumbles, gluten-free tortilla strips, and lime wedges. You can find Cotija cheese at most major grocery stores, but you can also substitute another crumbly cheese like feta.

CRISPY CORN FRITTERS

{ MAKES 6 FRITTERS }

 NF   **VT**

PREP TIME: 5 minutes

COOK TIME: 35 minutes

2 large eggs

½ teaspoon garlic powder

½ teaspoon onion powder

¼ teaspoon paprika

Pinch salt

Pinch freshly ground black pepper

1 (15-ounce) can sweet
corn, drained

½ cup All-Purpose Flour Blend
(page 171)

½ cup shredded sharp
cheddar cheese

¼ cup chopped scallions

¾ teaspoon baking powder

3 tablespoons unsalted butter

PRO TIP: After flipping the fritters,
use a spatula to press each one
into the skillet to flatten to a ½-inch
thickness. This is the optimal finger
food size (and it cuts down on
frying time).

For the longest time, I thought corn fritters
were the food version of a boring party. But a
few years ago, a friend introduced me to the real
version, which is quick-fried patties filled with
sweet corn kernels, creamy cheese, fragrant
scallions, and a combination of onion, garlic,
and paprika that delivers the most amazing
finger-food concoction known to humankind.
Who says you can't have fried finger foods with
all your friends? Bring it on!

1. In a medium bowl, combine the eggs, garlic
    powder, onion powder, paprika, salt, and
    pepper and beat together. Add the corn, flour
    blend, cheese, scallions, and baking powder
    and stir well.

2. Melt the butter in a large nonstick skillet
    over medium heat. Form the mixture into
    6 equal-size patties. Working in two batches,
    fry the patties for 12 to 15 minutes, until the
    bottoms are golden brown, then flip and fry for
    an additional 5 to 7 minutes, until both sides
    are golden brown.

3. Transfer the fritters onto a plate lined with
    paper towels to cool. Serve warm.

4. Store leftovers in an airtight container in the
    refrigerator for up to 4 days.

CLASSIC CORNBREAD MUFFINS

{ MAKES 12 MUFFINS }

PREP TIME: 15 minutes

COOK TIME: 15 minutes

1 cup gluten-free yellow cornmeal

1 cup coconut flour

½ teaspoon baking soda

½ teaspoon salt

1 cup buttermilk

½ cup unsalted butter, melted, plus more for serving

½ cup sugar

⅓ cup shredded cheddar cheese

2 large eggs

2 tablespoons honey, plus more for drizzling

There's no better partner to a warm, rich chili (like True Texas Chili, page 89) than a sweet, fluffy cornbread muffin. These muffins come together in just 30 minutes—the perfect side to your already perfect family meal.

1. Preheat the oven to 350°F. Lightly spray a 12-cup muffin tin with gluten-free cooking spray.

2. In a large bowl, combine the cornmeal, coconut flour, baking soda, and salt and mix to blend.

3. In another large bowl, mix together the buttermilk, butter, sugar, cheese, eggs, and honey. Pour the buttermilk mixture over the dry mixture and stir until thoroughly combined.

4. Fill the cups of the muffin tin equally with the batter. Bake for 14 to 18 minutes, or until the edges are lightly browned and a toothpick inserted into the center of a muffin comes out clean.

5. Store leftovers in an airtight container at room temperature for up to 3 days.

PRO TIP: Cornbread muffins are best served with a drizzle of honey over the top or with a pat of butter melted inside.

OLD-FASHIONED ONION RINGS

{ SERVES 4 }

PREP TIME: 10 minutes

COOK TIME: 15 minutes

Cooking oil, such as corn or canola

1½ cups white rice flour

2 teaspoons paprika

2 teaspoons freshly ground black pepper

1 teaspoon cayenne pepper

1 teaspoon garlic powder

Salt

1 large egg, beaten

1 cup buttermilk

3 tablespoons honey

2 tablespoons gluten-free sriracha

2 medium sweet onions, cut into ½-inch-thick rings

There is something joyful about onion rings. It could be the crunchy outer coating, so crisp and light, or the fragrant, tender centers. Or it could be that ring shape—so easy to pinch between fingers and dip into sauces and so fun to play with. (Don't pretend you've never put an onion ring on your finger.) A delicious snack for kids and adults alike, these onion rings are also easily customizable depending on your spice preferences.

1. Pour ½ to 1 inch of oil into a large skillet and set it over medium heat.

2. In a large bowl, combine the rice flour, paprika, black pepper, cayenne pepper, garlic powder, and salt to taste, mixing to blend. In another large bowl, mix together the egg, buttermilk, honey, and sriracha.

3. Test the oil by dropping a small bit of batter into it. If the batter sizzles immediately, the oil is hot enough to cook in. Dip each onion ring into the liquid egg mixture, allowing the excess to drip off, then dredge it in the flour mixture, coating the entire ring.

4. Cooking in batches, quickly place each ring in the hot oil and fry until it's golden brown, 1 to 3 minutes. Once golden, flip and fry the other side for an additional 1 to 3 minutes.

5. Use a slotted spoon or tongs to carefully remove the onion ring from the skillet and place on a baking sheet lined with paper towels to cool before serving.

6. Store leftovers in an airtight container in the refrigerator for up to 3 days.

PRO TIP: These onion rings have a touch of heat from the sriracha in the coating, so they pair nicely with creamy dips and dressings.

GOLDEN CORN SOUFFLÉ

{ SERVES 8 }

PREP TIME: 15 minutes

COOK TIME: 55 minutes

2 (15-ounce) cans whole kernel sweet corn

2 (15-ounce) cans gluten-free creamed corn

1 (8-ounce) package cream cheese, softened

2 cups shredded Swiss cheese

3 tablespoons unsalted butter, melted

¾ cup gluten-free corn flake cereal, crushed

Parsley, for garnish

Freshly ground black pepper, for garnish

PRO TIP: For easy crushing, place the corn flakes in a resealable plastic bag and press out the extra air. Use the bottom of a coffee mug to crush the cereal one section at a time, applying pressure while slowly twisting. Continue this press-and-twist maneuver until all the cereal is crushed.

Warm and gooey, cheesy and creamy, delicious sweet corn kernels topped with crunchy golden topping—do I have your attention yet? This golden corn soufflé promises all this and more. My family makes a double batch of this recipe for every major holiday, and we fight to see who can scoop the most onto their plate.

1. Preheat the oven to 375°F.

2. In a 9-by-13-inch baking dish, combine the corn, creamed corn, cream cheese, and Swiss cheese. Mix thoroughly.

3. Bake for 40 minutes.

4. In a small bowl, combine the butter and cereal, mixing well. Sprinkle on top of the baked corn mixture.

5. Place the baking dish back into the oven and cook for an additional 12 to 15 minutes, until the cereal topping is fragrant and turns golden brown.

6. Remove from the oven, garnish with parsley and pepper, and cool for 5 minutes to set. Serve warm.

7. Store leftovers in an airtight container in the refrigerator for up to 5 days.

SWEET POTATO HASH

{ SERVES 6 }

 DF NF V

PREP TIME: 10 minutes

COOK TIME: 40 minutes

1 large sweet potato, peeled and cubed

1 pound Brussels sprouts, trimmed and halved

1 cup corn kernels

¼ cup olive oil

2 tablespoons white wine vinegar

¾ teaspoon ground cumin

½ teaspoon garlic powder

¼ teaspoon freshly ground black pepper, plus more to taste

Salt

Need an easy side dish for a fall or winter meal? This recipe pairs soft pieces of sweet potato with a generous amount of sweet corn and crisp-tender Brussels sprouts, all sprinkled with a quick cumin-and-pepper spice mix.

1. Preheat the oven to 425°F. Line a rimmed baking sheet with aluminum foil.

2. In a large bowl, combine the sweet potato, Brussels sprouts, corn, oil, vinegar, cumin, garlic powder, and pepper and mix together. Spread the mixture in a single layer on the baking sheet.

3. Cook for 20 minutes, then remove from the oven and stir the vegetables. Cook for an additional 20 to 25 minutes, or until brown on the edges and fork-tender. Add salt and pepper to taste. Serve warm.

4. Store leftovers in an airtight container in the refrigerator for up to 3 days.

PRO TIP: Need to use up vegetables before they go bad? Feel free to customize. Swap out the Brussels sprouts for kale or bell pepper, or the corn for mushrooms, zucchini, or yellow squash. You can even replace the sweet potato with Yukon Gold or russet potatoes.

MASHED POTATOES AND GRAVY

{ SERVES 6 }

NF 30

PREP TIME: 15 minutes

COOK TIME: 15 minutes

2 pounds russet or yellow potatoes, halved

⅓ cup sour cream, plus ½ cup

3 tablespoons unsalted butter

1 cup gluten-free chicken stock

1 tablespoon Worcestershire sauce

1 teaspoon garlic powder

½ cup sliced mushrooms

1½ tablespoons cornstarch

Is there a side dish more classically comfort food than mashed potatoes and gravy? I don't think so. Mashed potatoes aren't necessarily a problem for gluten-free dieters, but the gravy can be. This recipe pulls a few simple ingredients together to create a thick, savory gluten-free gravy.

1. Put the potatoes in a large heavy-bottom pot or Dutch oven and cover them with water. Boil for 15 minutes, until fork-tender. Drain, mash the potatoes using a potato masher, and stir in the ⅓ cup of sour cream and butter until well combined.

2. In a medium saucepan, combine the chicken stock, Worcestershire sauce, and garlic powder over medium heat. Bring to a simmer. Add the mushrooms, the remaining ½ cup of sour cream, and cornstarch and stir to combine. Simmer for 3 to 4 minutes, until slightly thickened. Pour the gravy over the warm mashed potatoes and serve.

3. Store leftovers in an airtight container in the refrigerator for up to 3 days.

PRO TIP: You can use leftover mashed potatoes in Shepherd's Pie (page 141), Loaded Baked Potato Soup (page 87), or even Twice-Baked Potatoes (page 73).

TWICE-BAKED POTATOES

{ SERVES 6 }

NF

PREP TIME: 20 minutes

COOK TIME: 25 minutes

3 bacon slices

3 large russet potatoes

¾ cup shredded cheddar cheese

½ cup sour cream

3 scallions, diced

1 tablespoon olive oil

Salt

6 tablespoons Bread Crumbs
(page 170)

You've never seen a twice-baked potato quite like this. This method cuts the potatoes to create a crisp potato cup from which you can spoon out warm, cheesy bites of potato, cheese, bacon, and scallions.

1. In a large saucepan or Dutch oven, cook the bacon over medium heat to your desired doneness. Transfer to a plate lined with paper towels and let cool, then crumble.

2. Preheat the oven to 400°F. Poke the potatoes all over with a fork, then cook in the microwave for 8 minutes, flipping halfway through.

3. Once cool enough to handle, slice off the very ends of the potatoes so they can stand up, then slice the potatoes in half width-wise.

4. Carefully scoop out the insides of the potato halves, being careful not to scoop through the opposite end, and place the flesh in a medium bowl.

5. Mash the potato insides, then add the cheese, sour cream, bacon crumbles, and scallions. Coat the outside of each potato half with olive oil and salt to taste.

CONTINUED

6. Stand up the potato halves in a baking dish and fill the skins with the potato mixture. Sprinkle the bread crumbs on top. Bake for 15 to 20 minutes, or until warmed through.

7. Cool for 3 to 4 minutes before serving.

8. Store leftovers in an airtight container in the refrigerator for up to 3 days.

PRO TIP: Use an ice cream scoop to remove the flesh of the potato without accidentally puncturing the opposite end. It's easy to dig too deep with a regular spoon.

EASY HASH BROWN CASSEROLE

{ SERVES 8 }

PREP TIME: 10 minutes

COOK TIME: 55 minutes

1 pound frozen shredded hash browns

1 (10.5-ounce) can gluten-free cream of chicken soup (or Corn Chowder, page 86)

6 ounces cream cheese, room temperature

1 cup shredded cheddar or Colby Jack cheese

2 tablespoons unsalted butter, melted

½ teaspoon salt

1 cup Bread Crumbs (page 170)

Many people refer to this hash brown casserole as "funeral potatoes" because it's comforting enough to soothe a grieving heart. Whatever its name, this dish has been a staple in my family for decades. There's something so soul-warming about baked hash browns smothered in creamy layers with a garlicky crisp bread topping. Scoop after scoop, this dish becomes more and more addictive.

1. Preheat the oven to 375°F.

2. In a large bowl, combine the hash browns, soup, cream cheese, cheddar cheese, butter, and salt. Stir until well combined. Transfer the mixture to a 9-by-13-inch baking dish, and top with a thin, even layer of bread crumbs.

3. Bake for 55 minutes, or until the topping and edges are golden brown.

4. Cool for at least 5 minutes before serving.

5. Store leftovers in an airtight container in the refrigerator for up to 3 days.

PRO TIP: This dish is a huge hit at parties and gatherings. If you're planning to serve this to a large group, you'd better make plenty. Double all the ingredients except the bread crumbs and increase the bake time to 75 minutes.

ULTIMATE BAKED MAC AND CHEESE

{ SERVES 8 }

PREP TIME: 10 minutes

COOK TIME: 20 minutes

8 ounces elbow-shaped gluten-free pasta, such as Ancient Harvest Quinoa and Corn Blend

2½ tablespoons unsalted butter

2 tablespoons All-Purpose Flour Blend (page 171)

1¼ cups milk

2 teaspoons garlic powder

¼ teaspoon paprika

Salt

Freshly ground black pepper

4 ounces (½ package) cream cheese

1 cup shredded mozzarella cheese

1 cup shredded cheese, such as cheddar, Colby, or Jack

1 cup Bread Crumbs (page 170)

Macaroni and cheese—the gold standard of comfort food. There's nothing better than tender pasta smothered in homemade cheese sauce and baked with savory, crunchy topping. This dish comes out of the oven with a golden brown crust just ready to be devoured.

1. Preheat the oven to broil.

2. Fill a large saucepan halfway with water and bring to a boil. Add the pasta and cook for 4 minutes, then drain and run cold water over the pasta to stop it from cooking.

3. In a large oven-safe skillet, melt the butter over medium heat. Add the flour blend and stir continuously for 1 to 2 minutes, until clumpy and fragrant. Slowly add in the milk, stirring continuously, until even and creamy, 2 to 3 minutes.

4. Add the garlic powder, paprika, and salt and pepper to taste. Add the cream cheese and allow it to melt. Add the shredded cheeses and stir until just melted, about 2 minutes.

5. Pour the pasta into the skillet and stir just enough to evenly coat the pasta with the cheese sauce. Sprinkle the bread crumbs over the pasta. Broil for 2 to 3 minutes, or until the bread crumbs start to turn a deeper shade of golden brown. Cool for 2 to 3 minutes before serving.

6. Store leftovers in an airtight container in the refrigerator for up to 4 days.

PRO TIP: Be sure to stop cooking the pasta before it's fully cooked or the finished dish will be overdone and possibly mushy.

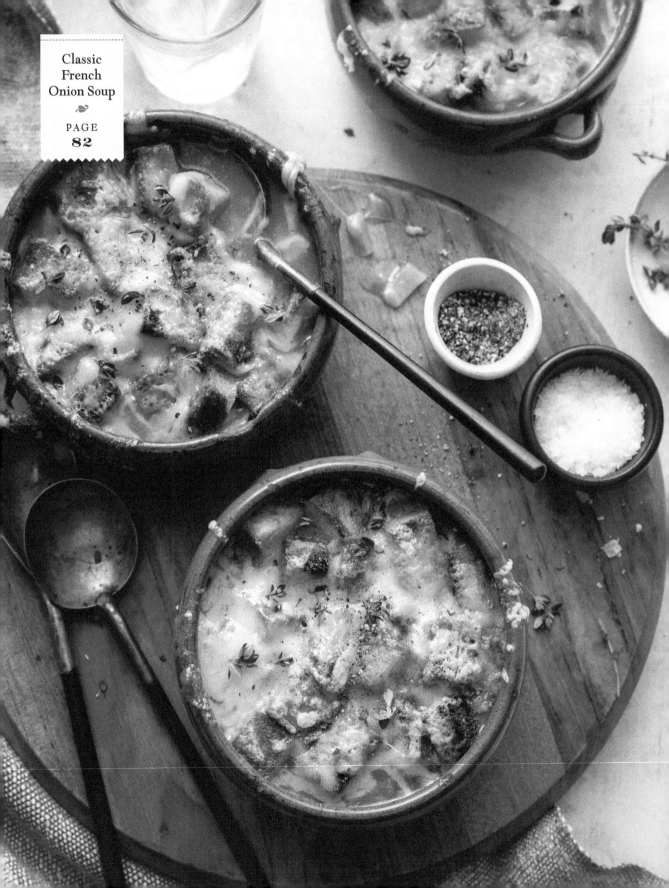

Classic
French
Onion Soup

PAGE
82

{ 05 }
SOUPS AND STEWS

EGG DROP SOUP

{ SERVES 4 }

DF NF 30

PREP TIME: 10 minutes

COOK TIME: 15 minutes

1 tablespoon cooking oil, such as olive, coconut, or canola

½ cup diced onion

5 cups gluten-free low-sodium chicken broth

2 large eggs

2 cups fresh baby spinach or kale

1½ tablespoons yellow mustard

1½ tablespoons rice vinegar

1 tablespoon gluten-free chili paste or sriracha

½ teaspoon red pepper flakes

¼ teaspoon ground ginger

⅛ teaspoon ground anise

Salt

Freshly ground black pepper

Scallions, diced, for garnish

If Chinese takeout is your comfort food of choice, try this egg drop soup. This recipe is protein-packed with spinach and simmered eggs, flavored with a kimchi-like sauce, and blended with quick rice noodles, all floating together in perfect delicious harmony.

1. In a large pot, heat the oil and onion over medium heat and cook, stirring occasionally, until golden brown and fragrant, about 2 minutes. Add the broth and heat until just simmering.

2. Beat the eggs, then slowly add them in with a fork (see pro tip). Add the spinach, and allow the soup to simmer and the spinach to wilt.

3. In a small bowl, mix the mustard, vinegar, chili paste, red pepper flakes, ginger, and anise. Once the spinach has wilted, add the sauce to the soup and stir. Add salt and pepper to taste. Serve warm topped with scallions.

4. Store leftovers in an airtight container in the refrigerator for up to 4 days.

PRO TIP: While the soup is barely simmering, use the prongs of a fork to slowly add in the beaten egg a little at a time. Quickly stir the egg after every forkful. It will cook through almost immediately in the warm soup. For some extra umami flavor, add ½ teaspoon of fish sauce.

CHICKEN NOODLE SOUP

{ SERVES 4 }

DF NF

PREP TIME: 15 minutes

COOK TIME: 35 minutes

2 medium boneless, skinless chicken breasts

2 tablespoons cooking oil, such as olive, coconut, or canola, plus more if needed

½ medium onion, chopped

2 teaspoons minced garlic

1 medium carrot, diced

2 teaspoons dried oregano

½ teaspoon salt

¼ teaspoon ground coriander

8 cups gluten-free low-sodium chicken broth

10 ounces gluten-free pasta of choice

PRO TIP: This soup is great to make in batches to freeze for later. Pack it up for college students or friends who need freezer meals. Transfer soup into freezer-safe plastic storage bags and freeze for up to 4 months. When ready to use, thaw in the refrigerator for 24 hours before reheating.

If there were a poster child for comfort foods, it would be chicken soup, which so many people turn to when under the weather or feeling blue. There is something about a warm broth with tender pieces of vegetable and chicken mixed together that makes any sore throat or burdened heart feel a little better.

1. Place the chicken in a large pot and fill with enough water to cover. Bring to a boil and boil the chicken until cooked through, 10 to 15 minutes, depending on the size. Drain and cool. When cool enough to handle, cut into cubes.

2. In a large pot, heat the oil over medium heat, then add the onion and garlic. Cook until brown, about 5 minutes.

3. Add the carrot, oregano, salt, and coriander and cook for 1 minute, stirring occasionally. If ingredients start to stick to the pan, add a bit more oil.

4. Add the broth and cooked chicken and bring to a boil. Add the noodles and cook according to package directions. Serve warm or hot.

5. Store leftovers in an airtight container in the refrigerator for up to 3 days.

CLASSIC FRENCH ONION SOUP

{ SERVES 4 }

NF

PREP TIME: 15 minutes

COOK TIME: 45 minutes

5⅓ tablespoons unsalted butter

1 tablespoon minced garlic

2 teaspoons packed light brown sugar

½ teaspoon salt

3 medium sweet onions, coarsely chopped

3 tablespoons All-Purpose Flour Blend (page 171)

4 cups gluten-free beef broth

1½ tablespoons Worcestershire sauce

10 thyme sprigs, plus 4 sprigs for garnish

1 cup grated or shredded Gruyère cheese

Want to impress your guests? A little herb garnish takes up any recipe a notch, but especially melty, cheesy dishes like this one. I like to show off the perfectly golden, gooey cheese topped with a sprig or two of fresh thyme. Your guests will be enchanted by this mouthwatering presentation.

1. In a large pot or Dutch oven, melt the butter over medium heat. Add the garlic, brown sugar, salt, and onions, stirring to coat the onions in the liquid. Allow the onions to soften, about 5 minutes, then reduce the heat to medium-low and cook for an additional 25 minutes.

2. Preheat the oven to broil.

3. Stir in the flour blend to coat the onions, then add the broth, 1 cup at a time, stirring for 10 to 15 seconds between each cup. Add the Worcestershire sauce and thyme. Allow the soup to come to a simmer. Cook, stirring occasionally, for 5 minutes, or until the soup starts to thicken slightly. Remove the thyme.

4. Pour the soup into oven-safe bowls, sprinkle with the Gruyère cheese, and broil for 2 to 3 minutes, or until the cheese has melted and the edges are turning golden brown. Cool for 2 to 3 minutes before serving, topped with a sprig of thyme.

5. Store leftovers in an airtight container in the refrigerator for up to 4 days.

PRO TIP: This soup is terrific with homemade gluten-free croutons (pictured on page 78). Chop 2 slices of Sandwich Bread (page 50) into 1-inch cubes, spray with gluten-free cooking spray, and sprinkle with garlic salt. Place the cubes on a nonstick baking sheet and broil, watching carefully, for 3 to 4 minutes, or until the edges start to toast. Flip and broil for an additional 3 to 4 minutes. Remove from the oven to cool. Sprinkle the croutons over the soup before adding the cheese in step 4. Store leftover croutons in an airtight container in the freezer for up to 6 months. Thaw at room temperature for 1 hour before reusing.

CREAMY CURRY SOUP
{ SERVES 4 }

DF NF 30

PREP TIME: 10 minutes

COOK TIME: 20 minutes

2 tablespoons oil, such as canola, coconut, or olive

1 tablespoon minced garlic

½ red onion, chopped

2 tablespoons gluten-free red Thai chili paste, such as Thai Kitchen brand

¼ teaspoon ground ginger

4 cups vegetable broth

1 (13-ounce) can full-fat coconut milk

1½ tablespoons fish sauce

1½ teaspoons packed light brown sugar

8 ounces gluten-free pad Thai noodles, such as Annie Chun's brand

2 cups fresh baby spinach

I am picky about my curry dishes, but this creamy soup is something special. The mellow aromas and flavors of red curry allow the flavorful base to shine through.

1. In a large saucepan, heat the oil over medium heat. Add the garlic and onion and cook for 1 minute, then add the chili paste and ginger, stir, and cook for an additional 1 minute.

2. Add the broth, bring to a simmer, and cook for 5 minutes. Add the coconut milk, fish sauce, and brown sugar and return to a simmer.

3. Add the pad Thai noodles and simmer for an additional 4 minutes, then add the spinach, stir, and simmer for 2 minutes, or until the spinach has wilted.

4. Remove from the heat. Ladle the soup into bowls and serve warm.

5. Store leftovers in an airtight container in the refrigerator for up to 4 days.

PRO TIP: To elevate this dish, garnish each bowl with a generous handful of chopped fresh cilantro leaves, freshly squeezed lime juice, a few extra finely chopped pieces of red onion, and a drizzle of gluten-free sriracha. The orange, green, and purple colors will dazzle your diners.

CHEESY ENCHILADA SOUP

{ SERVES 6 TO 8 }

NF 30

PREP TIME: 10 minutes

COOK TIME: 20 minutes

2 tablespoons cooking oil, such as olive, coconut, or canola

1 tablespoon minced garlic

½ sweet onion, chopped

1 pound ground beef

⅔ cup masa harina (corn flour)

2½ cups gluten-free low-sodium chicken or vegetable broth

3 (10-ounce) cans diced tomatoes and green chiles, such as Ro-Tel brand

1 (10-ounce) can gluten-free red enchilada sauce, such as Las Palmas brand

¾ teaspoon ground cumin

Salt

Freshly ground black pepper

2 cups shredded sharp cheddar cheese

Pico de gallo, for garnish

In 30 minutes, you can have a robust, cheesy soup with all the flavors of your favorite enchiladas.

1. In a large saucepan, heat the oil over medium heat. Add the garlic and onion, and cook until the onion is fragrant and translucent, 4 to 5 minutes. Add the ground beef and cook, stirring occasionally, until completely browned, 5 to 7 minutes.

2. Add the masa harina and cook for 1 minute, or until all the liquids have been absorbed. Immediately add the broth, tomatoes, enchilada sauce, cumin, and salt and pepper to taste.

3. Bring to a simmer, then cook for 5 minutes, stirring occasionally to prevent sticking.

4. Remove from the heat, add the cheese, and stir until melted and blended. Top with pico de gallo and serve warm.

5. Store leftovers in an airtight container in the refrigerator for up to 3 days.

PRO TIP: Enjoy this soup with salsa, sour cream, fresh cilantro, avocado slices, tortilla strips, or gluten-free sriracha. If you prefer to make it a dip, reduce the broth to ½ cup. Enjoy with tortilla chips, tortillas, or vegetable slices.

CORN CHOWDER

{ SERVES 6 }

NF

PREP TIME: 15 minutes

COOK TIME: 50 minutes

6 thick-cut or 8 regular bacon slices, diced

1 medium yellow onion, diced

2 teaspoons minced garlic

¼ cup All-Purpose Flour Blend (page 171)

4½ cups gluten-free low-sodium chicken broth

4 (15-ounce) cans sweet yellow corn, drained

1 pound russet or Yukon Gold potatoes, peeled and cut into ¼-inch-thick slices

½ teaspoon dried thyme

¼ teaspoon chili powder

Salt

Freshly ground black pepper

1½ cups heavy (whipping) cream

PRO TIP: This chowder is delicious on its own, but you can elevate its flavor profile even more by topping with chives or chopped scallions and a sprinkle of shredded cheddar cheese.

If you have a craving for a different kind of warm, hearty soup, try this corn chowder. This dish combines a creamy chicken broth with sweet, tender corn alongside soft potatoes and seasoning, all simmered together and topped with crisp bacon. What more comfort could your heart desire?

1. In a large saucepan or Dutch oven, cook the bacon over medium heat to your desired doneness. Transfer to a plate lined with paper towels and cool. Leave the bacon grease in the pan.

2. Add the onion and garlic and cook, stirring occasionally, about 5 minutes, until soft and translucent. Add the flour blend and cook about 1 minute, stirring continuously.

3. Pour in the broth while whisking, then bring to a simmer. Add the corn, potatoes, thyme, chili powder, and salt and pepper to taste. Return to a simmer. Continue cooking, stirring once every 5 minutes, for 20 to 25 minutes, until the potatoes are fork-tender.

4. Use an immersion blender or potato masher to blend the potatoes in the soup until smooth. Add the cream and return to a simmer.

5. Sprinkle with crumbled bacon and serve.

LOADED BAKED POTATO SOUP

{ SERVES 6 }

NF

PREP TIME: 10 minutes

COOK TIME: 52 minutes

3 tablespoons unsalted butter

½ large onion, chopped

2 teaspoons minced garlic

4 large russet potatoes, peeled and cubed

3 cups gluten-free low-sodium chicken broth

1½ teaspoons garlic powder

1 teaspoon salt

1 teaspoon freshly ground black pepper

1 cup milk

1 cup shredded cheddar cheese, plus more for garnish if desired

4 tablespoons diced scallions, plus more for garnish if desired

4 tablespoons bacon crumbles, plus more for garnish if desired

Need an easy soup to fill your belly and soul? This one combines hearty potatoes, garlic, and a sprinkle of bacon with a delightful spice mix that will leave everyone wanting more. You can also make a skinny version by using almond milk and cutting out half the cheese (but I'm betting you didn't come to this book looking for skinny recipes).

1. In a large pot or Dutch oven, melt the butter over medium heat. Add the onion and garlic and cook, stirring occasionally, until soft and fragrant, about 2 minutes. Add the potatoes, broth, garlic powder, salt, and pepper. Stir and bring to a simmer. Cook for 45 minutes.

2. Use an immersion blender or potato masher to mash the potatoes to your liking (see pro tip). Add the milk, cheese, scallions, and bacon crumbles. Stir to incorporate. Allow the cheese to melt, about 5 minutes.

3. Serve warm topped with extra cheese, scallions, and bacon crumbles, if desired.

4. Store leftovers in an airtight container in the refrigerator for up to 3 days.

PRO TIP: For a thicker, creamier soup, mash the potatoes more. If you like a more liquid soup with large chunks of potatoes, mash just a little.

BEER CHEESE SOUP

{ SERVES 4 }

NF

PREP TIME: 10 minutes

COOK TIME: 55 minutes

32 ounces gluten-free low-sodium chicken broth

12 ounces gluten-free beer

1½ tablespoons onion powder

1 tablespoon garlic powder

2 teaspoons minced garlic

1½ teaspoons Worcestershire sauce

½ teaspoon freshly ground black pepper

¼ teaspoon salt

3 cups shredded sharp cheddar cheese

½ cup heavy (whipping) cream

⅓ cup cornstarch

Gluten-free croutons, for garnish (see pro tip, page 83)

This beer cheese soup is so simple: just mix together a few ingredients and let it simmer. The combination of cheddar cheese, your favorite gluten-free beer, and tasty spices provides the base for this creamy, cheesy, inviting soup.

1. In a large pot or Dutch oven, combine the broth, beer, onion powder, garlic powder, garlic, Worcestershire sauce, pepper, and salt over medium heat. Bring to a simmer and cook for 30 minutes.

2. Stir in the cheese until melted and well blended. Stir in the cream and cornstarch, mixing thoroughly, and let cook for an additional 15 to 20 minutes.

3. If the cheese doesn't melt consistently, use a hand mixer or immersion blender to carefully blend to a thinner consistency. Serve topped with croutons.

4. Store leftovers in an airtight container in the refrigerator for up to 3 days.

PRO TIP: Other terrific garnishes include chopped scallions, bacon crumbles, or even popcorn. This cheesy soup is also fantastic with a kick of heat, so add 1 teaspoon of red pepper flakes, if desired. Want even more? A generous drizzle of gluten-free sriracha before serving will kick up the heat factor.

TRUE TEXAS CHILI

{ SERVES 6 TO 8 }

DF NF

PREP TIME: 10 minutes

COOK TIME: 1 hour

1 tablespoon cooking oil, such as olive, coconut, or canola

1 sweet onion, chopped

1 pound ground beef

1 (28-ounce) can diced tomatoes, with their juices

2 (14-ounce) cans tomato sauce

1 (4-ounce) can diced green chiles, with their juices

3 tablespoons chili powder

1 tablespoon sugar

1 teaspoon dried thyme

1 teaspoon dried oregano

1 teaspoon salt

This Texas chili comes from the kitchen of a true Southern momma who was born and raised in Texas. Texas chili differs from other chili in that it does not contain beans (*gasp*). Trust me, you won't miss them. You don't mess with Texas, and you don't dare mess with this recipe if you want to be authentic.

1. In a large saucepan or Dutch oven, heat the oil and onion over medium heat. Cook until fragrant and soft, about 4 minutes. Add the ground beef and cook, stirring occasionally, until completely browned, about 5 minutes.

2. Add the tomatoes with their juices, tomato sauce, chiles with their juices, chili powder, sugar, thyme, oregano, and salt and mix well. Cover and simmer for 50 minutes. Remove from the heat and serve warm (see pro tip for garnish ideas).

3. Store leftovers in an airtight container in the refrigerator for up to 3 days or in the freezer for up to 6 months.

PRO TIP: Garnish this hearty chili with sour cream, chives, and shredded cheddar cheese, if desired. This chili is amazing without beans, but if you are truly set in your chili ways, you can add a can of beans of your choice in step 2.

EASY BEEF STEW

{ SERVES 4 }

DF NF

PREP TIME: 10 minutes

COOK TIME: 2 hours, 10 minutes

1½ pounds beef stew meat, cubed

¼ cup All-Purpose Flour Blend
(page 171)

3 tablespoons olive oil

1 medium yellow or white onion,
roughly chopped

Salt

Freshly ground black pepper

3 cups gluten-free beef broth

1 (6-ounce) can tomato paste
with garlic

4 tablespoons
Worcestershire sauce

2½ teaspoons dried sage leaves

1½ tablespoons dried thyme

4 medium russet potatoes, cubed

2 cups frozen peas and carrots

This warming beef stew combines juicy pieces of
beef in a savory tomato-thyme broth with tender
pieces of potatoes and vegetables. It's perfect for
dipping crusty bread into.

1. Place the beef in a large resealable bag, add
   the flour blend, seal, and shake until the beef is
   coated in a light layer of flour.

2. In a Dutch oven, heat the oil over
   medium-high heat. Add the onion and
   cook until fragrant and slightly golden, 2 to
   3 minutes. Add the beef and cook, turning
   occasionally, until browned on all edges, about
   5 minutes. Sprinkle with a pinch of salt and
   pepper, if desired.

3. Add the broth, tomato paste, Worcestershire
   sauce, sage, and thyme. Stir to mix well, then
   bring to a boil. Reduce the heat to low and
   simmer, uncovered, for 1 hour.

4. Add the potatoes and peas and carrots, cover,
   and cook for an additional 1 hour. Serve warm.

5. Store leftovers in an airtight container in the
   refrigerator for up to 4 days.

PRO TIP: Look for beef chuck (the shoulder) or beef
round (the rump). For a more tender stew, after step 2,
combine all the ingredients in a slow cooker and cook
for 7 to 8 hours on low (recommended) or 3 to 4 hours
on high.

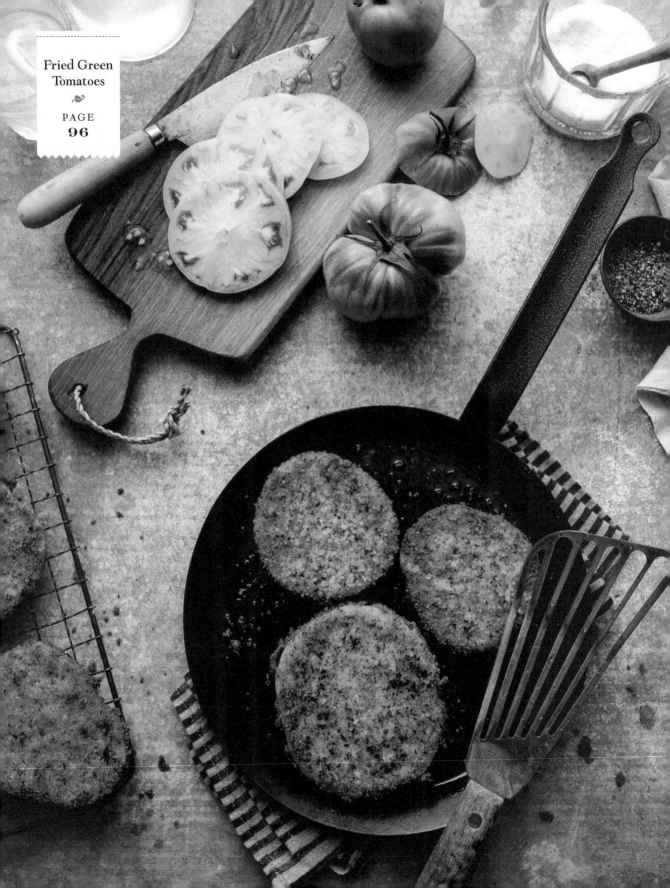

Fried Green
Tomatoes

PAGE
96

{ 06 }
SOUTHERN FAVORITES

CLASSIC HUSH PUPPIES

{ MAKES 18 HUSH PUPPIES }

PREP TIME: 15 minutes

COOK TIME: 15 minutes

Cooking oil, such as corn, vegetable, or canola

1 cup cornmeal

⅓ cup All-Purpose Flour Blend (page 171)

3 teaspoons sugar

1 teaspoon baking powder

½ teaspoon salt

¼ teaspoon baking soda

1 large egg, beaten

½ cup heavy (whipping) cream or buttermilk

PRO TIP: Want to mix it up a bit? Add ¼ cup of finely diced onion or jalapeño to the dough before frying. It'll add a fun, contrasting flavor punch.

Hush puppies are one of the most popular bite-size fried appetizers in the South. The crispy outer shell is balanced with a fluffy center made of cornmeal. Dip these in any spicy sauce or mayo-based dip for the perfect start to a meal or party.

1. Pour enough oil into a wok or large skillet to fill the bottom 1 inch deep. Heat over medium-low heat.

2. In a large bowl, combine the cornmeal, flour blend, sugar, baking powder, salt, and baking soda. Stir to combine. Add the egg and cream and stir to form a dough.

3. Use your hands to form ping pong–size dough balls. To test if the oil is hot enough, drop a small amount of batter into the oil. If the batter sizzles immediately, the oil is hot enough to cook in.

4. Carefully drop 3 to 5 dough balls into the oil and cook for 2 to 4 minutes, or until golden brown and crispy on the outside and cooked through on the inside.

5. Use an oil strainer or spatula to transfer the hush puppies to a cooling rack with a paper towel beneath it. Let cool slightly. Serve warm.

HOT CREAMED SPINACH

{ SERVES 4 }

NF   VT   30

PREP TIME: 10 minutes

COOK TIME: 15 minutes

2 tablespoons unsalted butter

1 tablespoon minced garlic

½ sweet onion, diced

⅓ cup milk

¼ cup heavy (whipping) cream

4 ounces (½ package)
cream cheese

¼ cup shredded Parmesan cheese

⅛ teaspoon ground nutmeg

⅛ teaspoon salt

1 (10-ounce) bag fresh
baby spinach

If the thought of wilted spinach in a creamy sauce doesn't seem very appetizing, it's because you've never had it this good. This recipe bathes fresh baby spinach leaves in a simmering mixture of garlic, cream, and cheese until the whole thing becomes warm and creamy. Technically, it's a vegetable dish, but you'd never know it from the rich, indulgent flavor.

1. In a large skillet, melt the butter over medium heat. Add the garlic and onion. Cook until fragrant and the onion is soft and translucent.

2. Add the milk, cream, cream cheese, Parmesan cheese, nutmeg, and salt and bring to a simmer.

3. Place heaping handfuls of the spinach into the simmering sauce, stir, and allow to wilt. Continue until all the spinach has wilted. Serve warm.

4. Store leftovers in an airtight container in the refrigerator for up to 2 days.

PRO TIP: Spinach shrinks a ton. Uncooked, it may look like a massive amount of greens, but once the spinach is wilted, this dish will be perfect for serving 4 to 6 people.

FRIED GREEN TOMATOES

{ SERVES 6 }

PREP TIME: 10 minutes

COOK TIME: 10 minutes

1 cup cooking oil, such as corn, vegetable, or canola

1 large unripe green tomato, cut into ¼-inch-thick slices

Salt

Freshly ground black pepper

½ cup All-Purpose Flour Blend (page 171)

1 teaspoon garlic powder

½ teaspoon onion powder

¼ teaspoon paprika

2 large eggs

1 tablespoon milk

1½ cups Bread Crumbs (page 170)

I was too much of a picky eater to try fried green tomatoes until I was well into adulthood, but now I'm kicking myself for not enjoying them my entire life. Crisp, juicy green tomato slices are seasoned and coated in a quick, tasty breading and fried to become the most delightful dish.

1. In a large skillet, heat the oil over medium-high heat. Season the tomato slices with salt and pepper.

2. In a medium bowl, stir together the flour, garlic powder, onion powder, and paprika. In another bowl, mix the eggs and milk. Put the bread crumbs in a third bowl.

3. Coat the tomato slices in the flour blend, then the egg mixture, allowing the excess to drip off. Place the tomato slices in the bread crumb bowl and press the bread crumbs carefully into each tomato.

4. Fry in batches, carefully lowering each breaded tomato into the hot oil. Fry for 1 to 2 minutes, until the breading starts to turn golden brown (see pro tip). Using a spatula, carefully flip and cook for an additional 1 to 2 minutes. Transfer each tomato to a plate lined with paper towels to cool and set. Serve warm.

5. Store leftovers in an airtight container in the refrigerator for up to 3 days.

PRO TIP: When you lower a tomato into the oil, it should begin sizzling immediately; if it does not, the oil isn't hot enough. To get the best results, make sure you let all the excess egg mixture drip off before adding the bread crumbs. Once you've pressed the bread crumbs into the tomato slice, slowly and carefully lift the slice out of the bowl so you don't knock any off before frying.

BISCUITS AND GRAVY BAKE

{ SERVES 8 }

PREP TIME: 20 minutes

COOK TIME: 45 minutes

FOR THE BISCUITS

¾ cup Biscuit Mix (page 172)

⅓ cup milk

2 tablespoons unsalted
butter, melted

1 large egg, beaten

FOR THE CASSEROLE

1 package cooked gluten-free
breakfast sausage crumbles, such
as Jimmy Dean or Butterball

6 large eggs

½ cup milk

½ cup shredded cheese, such as
Colby Jack

FOR THE GRAVY

2 tablespoons unsalted butter

4 tablespoons All-Purpose Flour
Blend (page 171)

1¾ cups gluten-free low-sodium
chicken broth

½ cup heavy (whipping) cream

Salt

Freshly ground black pepper

This bake is a big-batch version of that beloved Southern breakfast—biscuits and gravy. This recipe pairs fluffy breakfast biscuits with baked eggs and milk, sprinkles them with sausage crumbles, and smothers them in a rich, thick, creamy pepper gravy. After everything melts together in the oven, you're left with breakfast perfection, as well as a mouthwatering casserole you'll want to enjoy all day. This dish is a great idea for "breakfast for dinner" and delicious as leftovers, with the gravy soaking in and intensifying the flavor.

1. Preheat the oven to 375°F. Spray a 9-by-13-inch glass baking dish with gluten-free cooking spray.

2. **To make the biscuit dough:** In a medium bowl, mix together the biscuit mix, milk, butter, and egg. Spread evenly across the bottom of the baking dish.

3. **To make the casserole:** Spread the sausage crumbles in a single even layer over the biscuit dough. In a medium bowl, mix the eggs, milk, and cheese well, then pour over the dough and sausage.

4. **To make the gravy:** In a medium saucepan, melt the butter over medium heat. Add the flour blend and stir continuously for 30 seconds, until the liquids are fully absorbed. Add the broth ½ cup at a time, waiting until the gravy returns to a simmer before stirring and adding the next ½ cup. Add the cream and bring to a simmer. Add salt and pepper to taste and cook for 5 to 10 minutes. Remove from the heat and pour over the casserole.

5. Bake for 35 to 40 minutes, until the edges of the casserole are golden brown and bubbling. Remove from the heat and let it sit for 5 minutes before serving.

6. Store leftovers in an airtight container in the refrigerator for up to 3 days.

PRO TIP: If you don't have sausage crumbles, use any leftover cooked meats in the refrigerator. This bake is great with chicken, pork, and even steak.

SWEET POTATO CASSEROLE

{ SERVES 12 }

VT

PREP TIME: 15 minutes

COOK TIME: 45 minutes

5 large sweet potatoes

2 tablespoons unsalted butter, plus 2 tablespoons melted butter for the topping

1 cup packed light brown sugar, divided

2 large eggs

1½ teaspoons gluten-free vanilla extract

½ teaspoon salt

3½ tablespoons All-Purpose Flour Blend (page 171)

⅓ cup chopped pecans

3 cups gluten-free mini marshmallows

This is hands-down my family's favorite dish at a special holiday meal—sweet potatoes cooked up with butter, sugar, and spices and topped with sweetened nuts that will hook you in. The whole thing is topped with fluffy marshmallows. It's a sweet, smooth casserole that's perfect for any tableside celebration.

1. Preheat the oven to 350°F and set a rack in the center position. Spray an oven-safe 9-by-13-inch casserole dish with gluten-free cooking spray.

2. Poke the potatoes all over with a fork, set them on a large plate, and microwave on high for 9 minutes. Flip and microwave for an additional 9 minutes.

3. Cut each potato in half lengthwise and scoop out the insides, placing the flesh in a large bowl. While the potatoes are still hot, mash them with a potato masher, then add 2 tablespoons of butter, ½ cup of brown sugar, the eggs, vanilla, and salt and continue mashing until smooth and well combined. Spoon the mashed potatoes into the casserole dish.

4. In a small bowl, stir the flour, remaining ½ cup of brown sugar, pecans, and 2 tablespoons of melted butter until blended and crumbly. Sprinkle the topping over the mashed potatoes, then add the marshmallows in a single layer. Bake for 24 to 26 minutes, or until the top is lightly toasted. Cool for 2 to 3 minutes before serving.

5. Store leftovers in an airtight container in the refrigerator for up to 3 days.

PRO TIP: Elyon and Trader Joe's both make great gluten-free marshmallows. You can also buy them online or look up recipes to make your own.

FRIED CHICKEN AND WAFFLES

{ SERVES 6 }

NF

PREP TIME: 15 minutes

COOK TIME: 45 minutes

2 large eggs

3 tablespoons gluten-free powdered chicken seasoning

½ cup cornstarch

½ cup All-Purpose Flour Blend (page 171)

⅛ teaspoon salt

4 large boneless, skinless chicken breasts, cut into tenders

Cooking oil, such as peanut or canola

2 recipes Classic Waffles (page 23)

This chicken and waffles dish can't decide whether it wants to be breakfast, lunch, or dinner. There's no bad time to whip up a plate of fresh fried chicken nestled between fluffy waffles and drizzled with your favorite sweet finishes.

1. In a medium bowl, combine the eggs and chicken seasoning. Stir well.

2. In another medium bowl, mix together the cornstarch, flour, and salt.

3. Dredge each chicken tender in the egg mixture, coating all sides and allowing the excess to drip off. Place each tender in the flour mixture and flip until thoroughly coated. Place the tenders on a wire rack for 5 minutes.

4. Fill a deep frying pan or wok with enough oil to submerge the chicken pieces. Heat the oil to medium-high heat.

5. Drop 2 or 3 tenders into the oil and fry quickly. Cook for 5 to 8 minutes, until the chicken reaches an internal temperature of at least 165°F and the breading is a warm golden brown. Repeat in batches with the remaining tenders.

6.   Carefully transfer the cooked tenders to a wire rack with paper towels beneath it. Cool for 3 to 5 minutes. Divide the tenders into 6 equal portions and serve each portion on top of a fluffy waffle. Serve with a pat of butter and a hearty drizzle of syrup or honey.

7.   Store leftover chicken and waffles separately in airtight containers in the refrigerator for up to 3 days. Toast both briefly in the oven before serving again.

PRO TIP: If you prefer a bone-in cut of chicken (pictured), fry it for 5 to 7 minutes on each side. The internal temperature needs to reach 165°F before you remove it from the hot oil.

NASHVILLE HOT CHICKEN

{ SERVES 4 }

NF

PREP TIME: 10 minutes, plus 30 minutes to chill

COOK TIME: 45 minutes

½ cup buttermilk

¼ cup gluten-free hot sauce

4 skin-on chicken breasts

½ cup Biscuit Mix (page 172)

4 tablespoons gluten-free Cajun seasoning

3 tablespoons garlic powder

2 tablespoons cayenne pepper

2 tablespoons packed light brown sugar

¼ teaspoon salt

¼ teaspoon freshly ground black pepper

2 large eggs

¼ cup honey

2 tablespoons cooking oil, such as olive, coconut, or canola

Traditionally, this dish is deep-fried, but this incredible baked version is still crispy on the outside and oh-so-juicy on the inside. Don't worry: Just because this sweet and spicy Southern treat is a little healthier doesn't mean it's any less indulgent.

1. In a large bowl, combine the buttermilk and hot sauce, mixing thoroughly. Place the chicken breasts in the liquid, coating well. Cover the bowl in plastic wrap, and refrigerate for 30 to 60 minutes to marinate.

2. In a large bowl, combine the biscuit mix, Cajun seasoning, garlic powder, cayenne pepper, brown sugar, salt, and pepper. Mix well.

3. In a small bowl, whisk together the eggs and honey.

4. Preheat the oven to 400°F. Line a rimmed baking sheet with aluminum foil and place an oven-safe wire rack on top (if you have one).

5. In a large skillet, heat the oil over medium heat.

6. Dredge each breast in the egg mixture, allowing the excess to drip off. Coat thoroughly with the flour mixture.

7. Working in batches, place each breast in the hot skillet and cook until the outside is brown and crisp, 1 to 2 minutes on each side. Transfer the breasts to the wire rack on the lined baking sheet (or directly onto the sheet).

8. Bake for 20 to 30 minutes, or until the chicken is cooked through. Cool for about 5 minutes before serving.

9. Store leftover chicken in an airtight container in the refrigerator for up to 3 days.

SPICE IT UP: Want even more of a punch? Add 1 tablespoon of onion powder and ¼ teaspoon of ground cinnamon to the flour mix and a generous drizzle of gluten-free sriracha to the buttermilk marinade.

KING RANCH CHICKEN

{ SERVES 8 }

NF

PREP TIME: 15 minutes

COOK TIME: 50 minutes

1 (14.5-ounce) can gluten-free low-sodium chicken broth

1 (10.5-ounce) can gluten-free condensed cream of chicken soup

1 (10-ounce) can diced tomatoes and green chiles, such as Ro-Tel brand, with their juices

3 cups cubed chicken breast (about 1 pound)

2 cups shredded cheddar or Colby Jack cheese, plus more for sprinkling

½ red onion, chopped

Red pepper flakes or gluten-free sriracha (optional)

12 gluten-free corn tortillas

PRO TIP: If the corn tortillas are on the thinner side, double up when making the tortilla layers. This will help the tortillas stay intact and keep them from falling apart when serving.

Hearty and cheesy, this recipe is the epitome of comfort food. King ranch chicken is a creamy chicken enchilada casserole with a twist—it's served in lasagna form. It makes a wonderful weeknight dish to feast your eyes (and mouth) on.

1. Preheat the oven to 350°F.

2. In a large bowl, combine the broth, soup, tomatoes with their juices, chicken, cheese, onion, and red pepper flakes (if using). Stir to blend.

3. Arrange a single layer of tortillas on the bottom of a 9-by-13-inch baking dish. They will overlap a little.

4. Spread one-third of the mixture over the tortillas. Repeat this layering twice so there are 3 layers total, ending with the chicken mixture.

5. Sprinkle the top of the casserole with additional shredded cheese and bake for 50 to 60 minutes, or until the top is golden brown and the chicken pieces are cooked through. Let sit 5 minutes to cool and set before serving.

6. Store leftovers in an airtight container in the refrigerator for up to 3 days.

SOUTHERN SALISBURY STEAK

{ SERVES 6 }

DF NF

PREP TIME: 10 minutes

COOK TIME: 30 minutes

1 pound ground beef

½ medium green bell pepper, diced

½ cup Bread Crumbs (page 170)

1 large egg

3½ teaspoons ketchup, divided

2 teaspoons Worcestershire sauce, divided

1 teaspoon onion powder, divided

¼ teaspoon salt

1 teaspoon cooking oil, such as olive, coconut, or canola

2 tablespoons All-Purpose Flour Blend (page 171)

1½ cups gluten-free beef stock

1 cup chopped mushrooms

This Salisbury steak recipe is so easy and good. It's a one-pot recipe (yes, only one pot to clean up afterward), and it takes just minutes from start to finish. Everyone will be licking their plates clean of the savory gravy and tender, juicy beef patties.

1. In a large bowl, combine the ground beef, bell pepper, bread crumbs, egg, 2 teaspoons of ketchup, 1 teaspoon of Worcestershire sauce, ½ teaspoon of onion powder, and salt. Mix well.

2. In a large skillet, heat the oil over medium heat.

3. Using your hands, form the beef mixture into 9 equal-size patties. Working in three batches, place them in the hot skillet and brown for 4 minutes. Flip and brown for an additional 4 minutes on the other side, then transfer the patties to a plate. Reserve the juices in the pan.

CONTINUED ✍

4. In a small bowl, combine the remaining 1½ teaspoons of ketchup, remaining 1 teaspoon of Worcestershire sauce, remaining ½ teaspoon of onion powder, and the flour blend. Add the mixture to the juices in the hot skillet and stir for 1 minute. Add the stock and mushrooms, stir, and bring to a simmer. Cook for 5 to 7 minutes, or until the liquids start to thicken. Return the beef patties to the skillet and cook for 1 minute. Remove from the heat and serve immediately.

5. Store leftovers in an airtight container in the refrigerator for up to 3 days.

PRO TIP: Add some green to this dish by including halved Brussels sprouts, green beans, or broccoli florets to the cooking gravy with the mushrooms. This is just enough time to turn these vegetables into tender-crisp, gravy-simmered greens that go perfectly with the Salisbury steaks.

CHICKEN FRIED STEAK

{ SERVES 4 }

NF

PREP TIME: 15 minutes

COOK TIME: 35 minutes

FOR THE STEAKS

Cooking oil, such as corn, vegetable, or canola

3 large eggs

1½ cups All-Purpose Flour Blend (page 171)

1½ teaspoons garlic salt

1½ teaspoons paprika

1 teaspoon freshly ground black pepper

½ teaspoon onion powder

4 cubed steak patties (4 ounces each)

FOR THE GRAVY

2 tablespoons unsalted butter

4 tablespoons All-Purpose Flour Blend (page 171)

1¾ cups gluten-free low-sodium chicken broth

½ cup heavy (whipping) cream

Salt

Freshly ground black pepper

Despite the name, this dish is made with flavorful steak patties that are fried quickly to get a crisp, crunchy coating, then drizzled in a pepper gravy. This classic comfort food is so easy that even the most hesitant home chef can make it right in their own kitchen. This recipe makes a lot of pepper gravy, so feel free to smother the steaks, or save the extra for other delicious recipes (see pro tip).

1. Preheat the oven to 275°F. Pour ½ inch of oil into a large skillet and heat over medium heat.

2. **To make the steaks:** In a medium bowl, beat the eggs. In another medium bowl, combine the flour, garlic salt, paprika, black pepper, and onion powder. Mix well.

3. Place a steak patty in the flour mixture and coat all sides completely. Dredge the patty in the eggs, submerging it completely and allowing the excess to drip off. Place the patty back into the flour mixture, coating it all over once more.

4. Place the patty in the hot oil and cook for 4 minutes. Carefully flip and cook for an additional 4 to 5 minutes, or until cooked through.

CONTINUED ⋙

5. Repeat steps 3 and 4 with each remaining patty.

6. Transfer the patties onto a wire rack set over a paper towel or a large plate to catch the extra oil. Move the rack with the fried steaks onto a baking sheet and place in the warm oven while making the gravy.

7. **To make the gravy:** In a medium saucepan, melt the butter over medium heat. Add the flour and mix continuously for 30 seconds, until the liquids are fully absorbed. Add the broth ½ cup at a time, waiting until the gravy returns to a simmer before stirring and adding the next ½ cup. Repeat with the cream. Add salt and pepper to taste and cook for 5 to 10 minutes more. Remove from the heat. Serve the fried steaks warm with the gravy drizzled on top.

8. Store leftovers in an airtight container in the refrigerator for up to 3 days.

PRO TIP: This gravy is also terrific drizzled over cooked veggies, as a dipper for chicken tenders, or poured over cooked meats, such as turkey, chicken, or pork. If you'd like to make it dairy-free, substitute ¼ cup of gluten-free low-sodium chicken broth for the heavy cream.

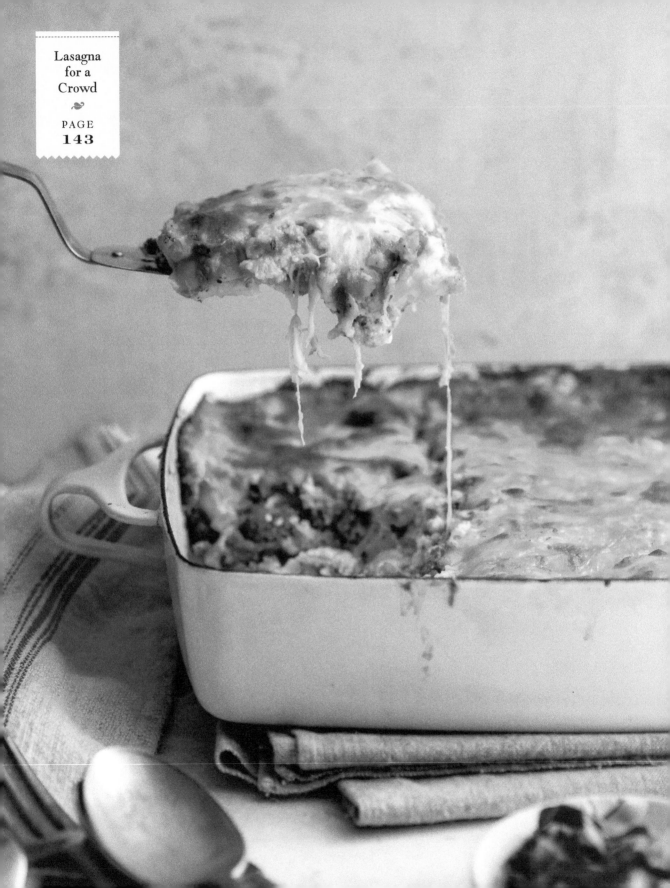

Lasagna
for a
Crowd

PAGE
143

{ 07 }
COMFORT FOOD CLASSICS

PEPPERONI PIZZA

{ SERVES 2 TO 4 }

NF 30

PREP TIME: 5 minutes

COOK TIME: 5 minutes

2 (10-inch) Thin Pizza Crusts, parbaked (page 44)

½ cup Spaghetti Sauce (page 173)

½ teaspoon garlic powder

2 cups shredded mozzarella cheese

2 tablespoons finely chopped fresh basil

Handful pepperoni slices

PRO TIP: Pizza crust is a blank canvas waiting for you to create your own culinary masterpiece. Make a white pie by swapping the sauce for ricotta, then add some fresh spinach. Load it up with veggies, meats, even breaded eggplant or chicken. Make it Hawaiian-style with pineapple and ham, or scampi-style with cooked shrimp, garlic, and butter—whatever warms you up inside.

This crisp, cheesy pepperoni pizza is my favorite way to end the workweek. From the easy-to-make homemade thin crust (which is perfectly crisp on the outside and soft on the inside), to the versatile spaghetti sauce (used here as pizza sauce), to the savory toppings, you'll love every single slice. Is it Friday yet?

1. Preheat the oven to 450°F and set a rack in the center position. Spray a large baking sheet with gluten-free cooking spray and place the pizza crusts on it. (Use two baking sheets if both crusts won't fit on one.)

2. Spread ¼ cup of spaghetti sauce in an even layer on top of each pizza crust, leaving 1 inch uncovered around the edge. Sprinkle ¼ teaspoon of garlic powder over the sauce on each pizza, followed by 1 cup of shredded cheese, 1 tablespoon of basil, and half the pepperoni.

3. Bake for 5 minutes, or until the cheese has melted and the crust is golden brown. Cool for 2 to 3 minutes before cutting into slices and serving.

4. Store leftovers in an airtight container or a plastic food-safe storage bag in the refrigerator for up to 3 days.

EASY FRIED RICE

{ SERVES 4 }

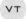

PREP TIME: 15 minutes

COOK TIME: 20 minutes

4 cups water

2 cups white rice

2 tablespoons sesame oil

1½ cups vegetables of choice

1 medium sweet onion, diced

3 garlic cloves, minced

4 scallions, chopped, plus more for garnish

2 large eggs

2 tablespoons gluten-free soy sauce or liquid aminos

Red pepper flakes (optional)

⅓ cup sliced almonds, for garnish

PRO TIP: Want to make this a meat-lover's fried rice? Stir in up to 1 pound of your preferred cooked protein when you add the rice in step 4.

What makes this fried rice so easy? For starters, it's done in about 30 minutes. It's also incredibly customizable. Mix in any vegetable or protein your heart desires (or your refrigerator contains—this recipe is a great way to use up whatever's just sitting there).

1. In a large saucepan, bring the water to a boil. Add the rice, stir, and cover. Return the water to a boil and cook for 10 to 15 minutes, or until the liquids are fully absorbed.

2. In a large skillet or wok, warm the sesame oil over medium-high heat. When it begins to shimmer, add the vegetables, onion, garlic, and scallions and cook for 3 minutes, until fragrant and beginning to brown.

3. Push the vegetable mixture to the sides of the skillet. Whisk the eggs in a small bowl, then add them to the center of the skillet. Cook, stirring frequently, until scrambled, about 2 minutes.

4. Add the rice to the skillet mixture, along with the soy sauce and red pepper flakes (if using). Mix well. Allow the juices to cook into the rice for 1 to 2 minutes before removing from the heat and sprinkling with scallions and almond slices and serving.

5. Store leftovers in an airtight container in the refrigerator for up to 5 days.

SAVORY MUSHROOM RISOTTO
{ SERVES 6 TO 8 }

 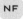

PREP TIME: 10 minutes

COOK TIME: 45 minutes

2 tablespoons unsalted butter

1 medium sweet onion, diced

1 tablespoon minced garlic

1 teaspoon freshly squeezed lemon juice

1½ tablespoons chopped fresh thyme

½ cup dry red wine

2 cups Arborio rice

1½ cups chopped mushrooms

6 cups vegetable broth

1 cup grated or shredded Parmesan cheese

Forget what you've heard about how risotto requires you to spend hours in the kitchen, stirring until your arms fall off. This recipe proves that you can make a creamy risotto in less than an hour.

1. In a large skillet, melt the butter over medium heat. Add the onion, garlic, lemon juice, and thyme and cook until fragrant, 3 to 4 minutes.

2. Add the wine and stir until the wine soaks into the onion and reduces, 4 to 5 minutes. Add the rice and stir to coat well. Add the mushrooms and stir to incorporate.

3. Add the broth ½ cup at a time, stirring to coat the rice well between each addition.

4. Once the broth is soaked in, use a fork to check the rice grains. Once tender, remove from the heat and serve immediately with a generous handful of Parmesan cheese over each bowl.

5. Store leftovers in an airtight container in the refrigerator for up to 5 days.

PRO TIP: You might be tempted to stir this dish continuously, but all you need is one good mix every time you add an additional ½ cup of broth. Sit back, relax, and pour yourself a little bit of that red wine. You deserve it—you conquered risotto.

CHICKEN TENDERS AND FRIES

{ SERVES 4 }

DF NF

PREP TIME: 15 minutes

COOK TIME: 55 minutes

FOR THE CHICKEN TENDERS

1 large egg, beaten

¼ cup All-Purpose Flour Blend (page 171)

1 cup Bread Crumbs (page 170)

2 large boneless, skinless chicken breasts, cut into tenders

FOR THE FRENCH FRIES

2 large russet potatoes, cut into fry-shaped sticks

3 teaspoons olive oil

¼ teaspoon salt or garlic salt

Cure those fast-food cravings right in your gluten-free kitchen. Juicy on the inside, crisp and golden on the outside, these chicken tenders are as delicious as their fast-food cousins and way healthier because they are baked. Tenders and fries are wonderful dipped in barbecue sauce, honey mustard, ranch dressing, or ketchup.

1. **To make the chicken tenders:** Preheat the oven to 400°F and line a baking sheet with aluminum foil. Lightly spray the foil with gluten-free cooking spray or brush with a light coat of olive oil.

2. In a small bowl, beat the egg. In another small bowl, place the flour blend. In a third small bowl, place the bread crumbs.

3. Using your hands, dip a chicken tender into the flour bowl, coating all over. Transfer the tender to the egg bowl and dredge thoroughly, allowing any excess egg to drip off. Dip directly in the bread crumbs bowl, pressing the bread crumbs into both sides. Place the tender on the baking sheet. Repeat with the remaining tenders.

4. Cook for 14 to 16 minutes, or until the tenders are golden brown and cooked through.

CONTINUED ↝

5. Store leftovers in an airtight container in the refrigerator for up to 3 days.

6. **To make the French fries:** Lay the sliced potato sticks on a large baking pan.

7. Drizzle with olive oil and use your hands or a silicone basting brush to coat the potatoes thoroughly.

8. Sprinkle with salt and mix again to distribute.

9. Bake at 400°F for 40 minutes, or until the fries are golden and crisp, flipping halfway through.

PRO TIP: Want this meal finished even faster? Bake the tenders and fries at the same time using two baking sheets. If you want a bit of heat to your chicken tenders, add ½ teaspoon of red pepper flakes to the bread crumbs.

HONEY MUSTARD CHICKEN

{ SERVES 4 }

DF NF

PREP TIME: 15 minutes

COOK TIME: 55 minutes

⅓ cup coconut oil, melted

2 large eggs

1½ cups cornstarch

1 tablespoon garlic powder

¼ teaspoon salt

¼ teaspoon freshly ground black pepper

1½ cups brown or white rice flour

1½ pounds boneless, skinless chicken breasts, cubed or sliced as tenders

¾ cup gluten-free barbecue sauce

4 tablespoons honey

3 tablespoons gluten-free Dijon mustard

½ tablespoon apple cider vinegar

This is an addictive, finger-licking, please-give-me-more recipe. Picture savory breaded chicken pieces, baked to perfection, and smothered in a sweet and tangy honey mustard sauce. Devour this at your local tailgate or a birthday party. Just be sure to bring plenty of napkins.

1. Preheat the oven to 350°F.

2. Spread the coconut oil in a 9-by-13-inch baking dish, distributing it evenly over the bottom of the dish.

3. In a medium bowl, beat the eggs.

4. In a large resealable bag, combine the cornstarch, garlic powder, salt, and pepper and mix well. In another large resealable bag, pour in the rice flour.

5. Dip the chicken pieces into the egg, allowing the excess to drip off. Working in batches, transfer the chicken to the bag with the rice flour, seal the bag, and shake until the chicken is evenly coated. Transfer the chicken pieces to the bag with the cornstarch mixture. Repeat the shaking technique.

CONTINUED

6. Place the coated chicken pieces in the baking dish and bake for 45 minutes, stirring every 15 minutes to allow the chicken to cook and crisp evenly.

7. In a medium bowl, combine the barbecue sauce, honey, mustard, and vinegar.

8. Pour the sauce over the top of the chicken, stirring to evenly coat.

9. Bake for an additional 10 minutes, or until the chicken is fully cooked and the sauce starts to thicken into a glaze. Serve warm. The sauce will thicken more while cooling.

10. Store leftovers in an airtight container in the refrigerator for up to 3 days.

PRO TIP: If you want a bit of heat, add ½ teaspoon of red pepper flakes to the sauce before pouring it over the chicken. Just before serving, add a drizzle of gluten-free sriracha on top.

CHICKEN PARMESAN

{ SERVES 4 }

NF

PREP TIME: 10 minutes

COOK TIME: 25 minutes

⅓ cup (5⅓ tablespoons) unsalted butter, melted

2 cups Bread Crumbs (page 170)

4 thin chicken breasts or 2 thick chicken breasts, halved horizontally

1 cup Spaghetti Sauce (page 173)

1 cup shredded mozzarella cheese

2 tablespoons fresh basil, chopped

Salt

Freshly ground black pepper

PRO TIP: Serve over gluten-free pasta, alongside your favorite steamed vegetables, or with a side of crusty French bread or Zucchini Bread (page 53).

This chicken Parmesan hits all the right notes for comfort food: The crunchy, garlicky breading turns to golden perfection, the red sauce captures the Italian spices, and the creamy mozzarella cheese strings goodness into every bite.

1. Preheat the oven to 425°F. Spray a baking sheet with gluten-free cooking spray.

2. In a small bowl, place the butter. In a second small bowl, place the bread crumbs.

3. Using your hands, dip a chicken breast into the butter, then into the bread crumbs, pressing the crumbs into the chicken. Place on the baking sheet. Repeat with the remaining chicken breasts. Bake for 22 minutes, until the chicken turns a darker shade of golden brown.

4. Remove from the oven. Over each breast, pour ¼ cup of spaghetti sauce, ¼ cup of mozzarella, and ½ tablespoon of basil. Return to the oven and broil for 1 to 2 minutes, or until the cheese has melted and the edges are starting to turn golden brown.

5. Remove from the heat, add salt and pepper to taste, and serve.

6. Store leftovers in an airtight container in the refrigerator for up to 3 days.

CHICKEN CORDON BLEU

{ SERVES 4 }

PREP TIME: 15 minutes

COOK TIME: 45 minutes

2 large eggs

1½ cups Bread Crumbs (page 170)

½ teaspoon garlic powder

¼ teaspoon onion powder

4 chicken breasts, cut
three-quarters of the way through
horizontally (hamburger-style)

4 slices ham

4 slices Swiss cheese or
8 tablespoons shredded

Chopped fresh parsley, for garnish

This gluten-free take on a classic is delicious and fun to make. The chicken is cut almost all the way through horizontally (like a hamburger bun), breaded, and cooked for a few minutes before you stuff it with juicy ham and Swiss cheese. You'll find the breaded chicken tender and warm, the ham savory-sweet, and the cheese delectably gooey. It's a thrill ride for your taste buds.

1. Preheat the oven to 350°F. Lightly spray a casserole dish with gluten-free cooking spray.

2. In a medium bowl, beat the eggs lightly with a fork. In another bowl, mix the bread crumbs, garlic powder, and onion powder.

3. Dip the chicken breasts into the beaten egg, allowing the excess to drip off. Press directly into the bread crumb mixture, making sure each piece is evenly coated.

4. Place the breaded chicken breasts, closed as if they were not cut, into the casserole dish, and bake for 15 minutes, until the breading turns a darker golden brown along the edges.

5. Carefully open each breast just enough to place one slice of ham and one slice of cheese (or 2 tablespoons of shredded cheese) inside. Press the chicken closed.

6. Bake the chicken breasts for an additional 30 to 35 minutes, or until cooked through. Serve hot, garnished with parsley.

7. Store leftovers in an airtight container in the refrigerator for up to 3 days.

PRO TIP: Enjoy playing around with this dish. Try stuffing each chicken breast with turkey and Swiss or bacon and cheddar for a modern, updated flavor.

CHICKEN CACCIATORE

{ SERVES 4 }

DF NF

PREP TIME: 10 minutes

COOK TIME: 50 minutes

2 tablespoons olive oil

4 boneless, skinless chicken breasts

2 tablespoons minced garlic

1 yellow onion, diced

1 cup sliced mushrooms

¾ cup pitted black olives

10 thyme sprigs

3 tablespoons chopped fresh basil

1 teaspoon dried oregano

½ cup dry red wine

2 (14-ounce) cans diced tomatoes with basil, garlic, and oregano

This chicken cacciatore will bring the rustic countryside feelings of yesteryear into your kitchen. The ingredients might be simple, but you'll want more of this mouthwatering chicken smothered in tomatoes, olives, and thyme sauce.

1. In a large skillet, warm the oil over medium-high heat until it begins to simmer. Add the chicken and garlic and cook for 10 minutes, flipping halfway, until both sides of the chicken have browned.

2. Add the onion, mushrooms, olives, thyme, basil, oregano, wine, and tomatoes over the top of the chicken and stir until thoroughly mixed.

3. Reduce the heat to medium and cook for 40 to 45 minutes, stirring occasionally, or until the chicken is fully cooked and falls apart. Remove the thyme before serving.

4. Store leftovers in an airtight container in the refrigerator for up to 3 days.

PRO TIP: Enjoy this cacciatore over gluten-free pasta, rice, quinoa, cauliflower rice, or sautéed vegetables.

CHICKEN POPPY SEED CASSEROLE

{ SERVES 4 }

PREP TIME: 15 minutes

COOK TIME: 30 minutes

2 tablespoons cooking oil, such as olive, coconut, or canola

3 boneless, skinless chicken breasts, cubed

2 tablespoons unsalted butter, plus 2 tablespoons melted butter

2 teaspoons minced garlic

4 tablespoons almond flour

¾ cup plain almond milk

¾ cup plain nonfat Greek yogurt

½ cup gluten-free low-sodium chicken broth

1 tablespoon poppy seeds

½ teaspoon freshly ground black pepper

¼ teaspoon salt

3 cups broccoli florets

1 cup Bread Crumbs (page 170)

As a kid, whenever I went to Grandma's house, she always put a creamy casserole on the dinner table for me to drool over. I have the fondest memories of her serving up large helpings of this chicken poppy seed casserole while the family talked and laughed about the latest happenings. I hope it brings you just as much nostalgia.

1. Preheat the oven to 375°F. Spray a 9-by-13-inch baking dish with gluten-free cooking spray.

2. In a large skillet, warm the oil over medium heat until shimmering. Add the chicken and cook for about 5 minutes, stirring occasionally, until browned but not yet cooked through. Remove from the heat.

3. In a medium saucepan, heat 2 tablespoons of butter over medium heat until melted. Add the garlic and cook until fragrant and starting to brown, about 2 minutes. Add the almond flour and mix until very clumpy, then slowly add the almond milk, stirring continuously, until smooth.

4. Add the yogurt, broth, poppy seeds, pepper, and salt. Cook, stirring occasionally, for 5 to 7 minutes. The sauce will start to bubble and thicken. Add the chicken and broccoli and stir to coat.

CONTINUED ✎

5. Transfer the mixture to the baking dish and top with bread crumbs. Drizzle the 2 tablespoons of melted butter over the bread crumbs and bake for 15 minutes, or until the top of the casserole is golden brown and the broccoli is cooked to your liking. Serve immediately.

6. Store leftovers in an airtight container in the refrigerator for up to 4 days.

PRO TIP: Not sure what else to do with poppy seeds? Sprinkle them over a steamy soup or on top of your favorite salad. If you don't have gluten-free bread crumbs on hand, you can use crushed gluten-free crackers for the crunchy golden topping. Even crushed gluten-free cereal would work in a pinch (and a hint of sweet from the cereal is a pleasant surprise for your palate).

SAUSAGE AND RICE STUFFED PEPPERS

{ SERVES 4 }

NF

PREP TIME: 15 minutes

COOK TIME: 45 minutes

5 medium red, yellow, or green bell peppers (see pro tip)

3 cups water

1½ cups white jasmine rice

1 pound gluten-free ground pork, chicken, or turkey (regular or spicy)

1½ cups chopped yellow onion

2 teaspoons minced garlic

¾ teaspoon gluten-free creole seasoning, plus more for garnish

¼ teaspoon freshly ground black pepper

¼ cup chopped scallions, plus more for garnish

4 tablespoons grated Parmesan cheese

As my family has discovered, there are about 101 ways to eat these peppers. Whether you like to start with the golden cheesy top, cut the pepper into bite-size pieces, or spoon out the savory rice mix, you will enjoy every single morsel of this dish. Resist the urge to lick your plate clean—or don't.

1. Preheat the oven to 400°F.

2. Cut the tops off 4 bell peppers. Using a paring knife or spoon, remove the seeds and ribs inside the peppers. Dice the fifth bell pepper, discarding the stem, seeds, and ribs. Measure ¾ cup of the diced bell pepper. Save the rest for a future dish.

3. In a 9-inch square baking dish, pour ¼ inch of water, then add the bell peppers, with the open tops facing upward. Bake for 10 minutes while you make the filling. This helps the peppers tenderize without becoming too crispy.

4. In a large saucepan, bring the water to a boil. Add the rice, stir, and cover. Reduce the heat to a simmer and cook for 10 to 15 minutes, or until the rice has absorbed all the water.

CONTINUED ✒

5. In a large skillet over medium-high heat, cook the pork, stirring frequently, for 5 minutes, until browned but not quite fully cooked. Add the onion and diced bell pepper. Cook for an additional 3 minutes, until the vegetables start to soften.

6. Add the garlic and cook for 1 minute. Add the rice and mix well, then add the creole seasoning and black pepper.

7. Remove from the heat and add the scallions. Mix well. Remove the bell peppers from the oven. Divide the rice mixture equally among the peppers, filling each generously.

8. Top each stuffed pepper with 1 tablespoon of Parmesan cheese and garnish with a bit of extra creole seasoning. Bake for 25 to 30 minutes, or until the cheesy tops turn golden brown.

9. Remove from the oven, sprinkle with an extra pinch of chopped scallions, and cool for 2 to 3 minutes before serving.

10. Store leftovers in an airtight container in the refrigerator for up to 3 days.

PRO TIP: To ensure the bell peppers will stand upright while cooking, look for those with four lobes on the bottom, rather than three.

SWEET AND SOUR PORK

{ SERVES 4 }

DF NF

PREP TIME: 15 minutes

COOK TIME: 55 minutes

⅓ cup coconut oil, melted

2 large eggs

1½ cups cornstarch

1 tablespoon plus 1½ teaspoons garlic powder, divided

¼ teaspoon salt

¼ teaspoon freshly ground black pepper

1½ cups brown or white rice flour

1½ pounds pork tenderloin, cubed

7 tablespoons gluten-free sweet chili paste

1 cup granulated sugar or coconut sugar

⅓ cup apple cider vinegar

3 tablespoons gluten-free soy sauce

Can't get that craving for Chinese takeout to go away? Feed it instead. This recipe tosses juicy pork in a gluten-free coating and bakes it to golden perfection. Pair this dish with a bed of steamed broccoli or fluffy rice, or even some Easy Fried Rice (page 115).

1. Preheat the oven to 350°F. Spread the coconut oil in a 9-by-13-inch baking dish, distributing evenly over the bottom of the dish.

2. In a medium bowl, beat the eggs lightly with a fork.

3. In a large resealable bag, combine the cornstarch, 1 tablespoon of garlic powder, salt, and pepper and shake to mix. In another large bag, pour the rice flour.

4. Working in batches, dip the pork pieces into the egg, allowing the excess to drip off. Then place the pork pieces into the bag with the flour, seal tightly, and shake the contents until evenly covered in flour. Transfer the pieces to the bag with the cornstarch mixture and repeat the shaking technique.

CONTINUED ᕦ

5. Place the coated pork pieces into the baking dish and bake for 45 minutes, stirring every 15 minutes to allow the pork to cook and crisp evenly.

6. In a medium bowl, combine the sweet chili paste, sugar, vinegar, soy sauce, and remaining 1½ teaspoons of garlic powder. Mix well.

7. Remove the pork from the oven and pour the sauce over the top, stirring to coat.

8. Return to the oven and bake for an additional 10 minutes, or until the pork is fully cooked and the sauce starts to thicken into a glaze.

9. Remove from the oven and cool slightly before serving. The sauce will continue to thicken while cooling.

10. Store leftovers in an airtight container in the refrigerator for up to 3 days.

PRO TIP: If you want a bit of heat, add ½ teaspoon of red pepper flakes to the sauce before pouring it over the pork. And just before serving, add a drizzle of gluten-free sriracha on top.

PORK CHOPS AND GRAVY

{ SERVES 4 }

NF

PREP TIME: 10 minutes

COOK TIME: 25 minutes

2 tablespoons coconut oil or olive oil

1 teaspoon minced garlic

4 boneless pork chops

¼ teaspoon garlic powder

¼ teaspoon freshly ground black pepper

4 tablespoons unsalted butter

4 tablespoons cornstarch or gluten-free flour of choice

1 cup gluten-free low-sodium chicken broth

1 tablespoon finely chopped fresh thyme

2 tablespoons plain nonfat Greek yogurt

Want an easy and quick meal ready in about 30 minutes, but one that tastes like you've been slaving away in the kitchen for hours? This is it! Pork chops are seasoned, sizzled in a skillet, and drizzled with a simple broth-based gravy that thickens to perfection in minutes. This dish is best served hot and steamy, alongside your family's favorite vegetables or cooked potato of choice.

1. In a large skillet, heat the oil over medium heat until it begins to shimmer. Add the garlic and stir occasionally until fragrant and golden brown, 1 to 2 minutes.

2. Sprinkle each side of the pork chops with the garlic powder and pepper. Place them in the pan. Sear on each side for 3 to 6 minutes, depending on thickness, until golden brown and fully cooked to an internal temperature of at least 145°F. Set aside to rest.

3. Reduce the heat to medium-low and melt the butter. Add the cornstarch and stir vigorously, until smooth. Add the broth and thyme, increase the heat to medium, and stir until smooth again. Allow the gravy to heat and thicken, about 5 minutes.

CONTINUED

4. Add the Greek yogurt and stir to melt into the gravy. Drizzle the gravy over the pork chops.

5. Store leftovers in an airtight container in the refrigerator for up to 3 days.

PRO TIP: When you shop for pork chops, choose ones that are pink versus pale and have a little marbling; they will be more flavorful. And if you prefer mushroom gravy, add ½ cup of your favorite chopped mushrooms to the skillet with the broth and thyme. The mushrooms will soften and give an earthy note to the gravy.

CLASSIC JAMBALAYA

{ SERVES 8 }

NF

PREP TIME: 15 minutes

COOK TIME: 35 minutes

2 tablespoons olive oil or butter

1 pound boneless, skinless chicken breasts, cubed

½ pound Andouille sausage links, cut into coins

1 cup diced onion

1 cup diced celery

1 cup diced red, yellow, or orange bell pepper

3 tablespoons gluten-free Cajun seasoning

4 cups gluten-free chicken stock

1 (14.5-ounce) can diced tomatoes, with juice

1 (6-ounce) can tomato paste

2 tablespoons Worcestershire sauce

2½ cups uncooked white rice

PRO TIP: The combination of diced onion, celery, and bell pepper is called the "holy trinity" of Cajun cooking.

Jambalaya is a casserole with roots in Louisiana. This one-pot sensation simmers meats of different kinds—usually sausage, shrimp, and chicken—with rice in a broth until the rice absorbs all the savory liquid. This dish will not only give you Cajun street cred, but also only one pan to clean.

1. In a large skillet or Dutch oven, warm the oil over medium heat. Add the chicken and cook until browned, about 5 minutes. Add the sausage and cook until browned, about 3 minutes.

2. Add the onion, celery, and bell pepper and cook, stirring occasionally, until the vegetables soften, about 3 minutes. Add the Cajun seasoning, stock, tomatoes with juice, tomato paste, Worcestershire sauce, and rice and mix thoroughly.

3. Cover and simmer, stirring occasionally, for 20 to 25 minutes, or until just a few tablespoons of liquid remain in the pan.

4. Remove from the heat and rest, covered, for 5 minutes. Uncover, stir, and serve.

5. Store leftovers in an airtight container in the refrigerator for up to 4 days. (This dish actually tends to taste better after a night in the refrigerator, as the flavors will intensify.)

HEARTY SLOPPY JOES

{ SERVES 4 }

NF 30

PREP TIME: 10 minutes

COOK TIME: 15 minutes

1 pound ground beef

½ sweet onion, diced

1 medium bell pepper, stemmed, seeded, and ribbed, diced

1½ cups gluten-free ketchup

¾ cup yellow mustard

4 tablespoons packed light brown sugar

4 toasted gluten-free burger buns or lettuce cups

1¼ cups shredded cheddar or Colby Jack cheese, divided, plus more for garnish

⅛ cup chopped scallions, plus more for garnish

PRO TIP: Prefer a Spicy Joe? Add red pepper flakes to taste or a splash of gluten-free sriracha while simmering the sauce.

This recipe helped me rekindle my long-lost love of Sloppy Joes after I became gluten-free. I missed the special combination of warm ground beef and savory sautéed onions and peppers, all smothered in a rich, tangy sauce and sandwiched between two buns. Fair warning: These are true to their name, so you'll want lots of napkins and maybe even a fork to scoop up what falls from your sandwich—it's too delicious not to eat every single morsel.

1. In a large skillet, cook the ground beef for 5 minutes over medium heat, stirring frequently, until it begins to brown. Drain off any excess grease. Add the onion and bell pepper and cook until the vegetables become tender and fragrant, an additional 2 to 3 minutes.

2. In a large bowl, combine the ketchup, mustard, and brown sugar and mix thoroughly. Add the sauce to the skillet, mix well, and simmer for 3 to 4 minutes. Remove from the heat.

3. Divide the sloppy joe meat equally among the buns or lettuce cups, top with cheese and scallions, and serve.

4. Store leftovers in an airtight container in the refrigerator for up to 5 days.

MARINARA MEATBALLS

{ MAKES 24 MEATBALLS }

DF NF 30

PREP TIME: 15 minutes

COOK TIME: 15 minutes

1 pound ground beef

1 large egg, beaten

1 tablespoon finely chopped
yellow onion

1¼ teaspoons liquid aminos,
coconut aminos, or gluten-free
soy sauce

½ teaspoon minced garlic

¼ teaspoon coarse salt

¼ teaspoon freshly ground
black pepper

1½ cups Spaghetti Sauce
(page 173)

PRO TIP: Want to make
perfect-size meatballs? Use an ice
cream scoop to portion out the
beef mixture into 24 equal-size
balls. If you don't have a mini
muffin tin, you can use a regular
muffin tin, but the meatballs will
not be as round.

Ah, meatballs. Another great recipe to get the
kids involved in, because what little one doesn't
like working with their hands (and, more
important, getting a little messy)? The drizzle
of homemade marinara after baking gives these
meatballs an extra layer of cozy heartiness.

1. Preheat the oven to 400°F.

2. In a large bowl, combine the ground beef, egg,
   onion, aminos, garlic, salt, and pepper and mix
   thoroughly with your hands.

3. Roll the beef mixture into 24 (1- to 1½-inch-
   thick) balls, and place each in a cup of a 24-cup
   mini muffin tin.

4. Bake for 10 minutes, use tongs to flip each
   meatball, and bake for an additional 5 minutes,
   or until the meatballs are thoroughly cooked
   and the outsides are nicely browned.

5. Carefully transfer the hot meatballs onto a
   plate lined with paper towels. Serve warm,
   drizzled with warm spaghetti sauce.

6. Store leftovers in an airtight container in the
   refrigerator for up to 3 days.

SOUTHERN GOULASH

{ SERVES 4 }

DF NF 30

PREP TIME: 10 minutes

COOK TIME: 15 minutes

8 ounces gluten-free pasta noodles

1½ pounds ground beef

2 (14-ounce) cans stewed or diced tomatoes

2 tablespoons dried chopped onion

¾ teaspoon freshly ground black pepper

½ teaspoon red pepper flakes (optional)

¼ teaspoon garlic powder

This 25-minute Southern Goulash is so simple, but the flavors will blow your mind with its savory tomatoes and ground beef simmered with pasta and herbs and sprinkled with garlic. I like to think of it as the homemade grown-up version of Hamburger Helper. If you like, take this dish up a notch by making it hot and spicy.

1. Cook the pasta according to package directions until al dente (tender but still firm), usually 4 to 5 minutes. Drain.

2. In a large skillet, brown the meat, stirring occasionally, over high heat until fully cooked, about 5 minutes. Drain the grease.

3. Add the pasta and mix thoroughly. Add the tomatoes, onion, black pepper, red pepper flakes (if using), and garlic powder.

4. Reduce the heat to medium-low and simmer, stirring occasionally, until the liquids start to evaporate, 3 to 4 minutes. Remove from the heat and serve.

5. Store leftovers in an airtight container in the refrigerator for up to 5 days.

PRO TIP: Gluten-free noodles are easy to overcook and can become mushy quickly. Check the pasta regularly while it's cooking and stop when it reaches an al dente consistency. If you cook it until fully soft, it will fall apart when you stir all the ingredients together.

BEEF STROGANOFF

{ SERVES 4 }

NF

PREP TIME: 10 minutes

COOK TIME: 25 minutes

4 tablespoons olive oil

1½ tablespoons minced garlic

1 cup diced sweet onion

1 cup chopped mushrooms

1 pound beef tips

1½ teaspoons paprika

6 tablespoons All-Purpose Flour Blend (page 171), divided

3½ cups gluten-free beef broth

2 teaspoons Worcestershire sauce

8 ounces gluten-free rotini pasta

1 cup sour cream

Salt

Freshly ground black pepper

When it comes to comfort foods involving pasta, this beef stroganoff is top dog. You'll want to serve this half pasta dish, half creamy soup delicacy in bowls with utensils that allow for the most slurping possible. Present this dish with steamed greens or crusty bread.

1. In a large skillet, heat the oil over medium heat. Add the garlic and cook, stirring occasionally, until fragrant and golden brown, 1 to 2 minutes.

2. Add the onion and mushrooms and cook, stirring occasionally, until fragrant and soft, 3 to 4 minutes. Add the beef and cook until thoroughly browned, 5 to 7 minutes. Sprinkle with the paprika and 3 tablespoons of flour blend and stir for 30 seconds to thicken.

3. Add the broth and Worcestershire sauce and bring to a simmer. Add the pasta and cook until the pasta is just becoming al dente.

CONTINUED ✎

4. Stir in the sour cream and remaining 3 tablespoons of flour and simmer for an additional 2 minutes. Remove from the heat and cool for 5 minutes. Season with salt and pepper.

5. Store leftovers in an airtight container in the refrigerator for up to 3 days.

PRO TIP: Gluten-free pastas are notorious for becoming mushy and grainy when overcooked. Check the pasta regularly until it's just becoming soft, then remove from the heat immediately. The noodles will continue to cook in the stroganoff sauce. I recommend Ancient Harvest Rotini Corn and Quinoa Pasta, because corn- and quinoa-based pastas tend to more of the classic pasta texture than rice-based pasta.

SKILLET BEEF POTPIE
{ SERVES 6 TO 8 }

NF

PREP TIME: 15 minutes

COOK TIME: 40 minutes

5 tablespoons unsalted butter, plus 4 tablespoons melted butter

1 pound ground beef

1 teaspoon minced garlic

1½ cups Biscuit Mix (page 172)

1 large egg, beaten

1⅔ cups heavy (whipping) cream, divided

2½ cups beef broth

1 teaspoon garlic salt

½ teaspoon freshly ground black pepper

1½ cups frozen vegetable mix

⅓ cup All-Purpose Flour Blend (page 171), plus more for dusting

This beef potpie is full of delicious layers and, dare I say, delicious secrets. Each bite packs a punch of hearty flavors, all sealed in a fluffy crust. This incredible dish is so easy to put together, and you can adapt it for those with sensitivities to nuts or dairy. No one will be able to resist.

1. Preheat the oven to 375°F.

2. In a large oven-safe skillet or Dutch oven, melt 5 tablespoons of butter over medium heat. Add the ground beef and garlic, and cook until browned, about 5 minutes.

3. In a large bowl, combine the biscuit mix, egg, 4 tablespoons of melted butter, and ⅔ cup of cream and stir until well blended.

4. To the skillet, add the broth, garlic salt, and pepper. Bring to a simmer and cook, 4 to 5 minutes. Add the remaining 1 cup of cream and frozen vegetables. Return to a simmer. Whisk in the flour blend and cook for 2 minutes.

CONTINUED ❧

5. Turn the dough onto a flat floured surface, and use your hands or a rolling pin to flatten it into a circle, about ¼ inch thick. Carefully lift the dough and lay it over the skillet, tucking in the sides. Bake for 25 minutes, then broil for 2 minutes, until the crust is a deep golden color. Cool for 5 minutes before serving.

6. Store leftovers in an airtight container in the refrigerator for up to 3 days.

PRO TIP: Want this dish to cook even more quickly? Use precooked ground beef or frozen grilled beef strips.

SHEPHERD'S PIE

{ SERVES 4 TO 6 }

NF

PREP TIME: 15 minutes

COOK TIME: 55 minutes

4 large or 6 medium
russet potatoes

5 tablespoons unsalted
butter, divided

1 medium sweet onion, diced

1 tablespoon minced garlic

1½ pounds ground beef

1 large carrot, cut into thin slices

3 teaspoons dried thyme

1 (15-ounce) can sweet
corn, drained

1 cup frozen peas

¾ cup sour cream

A delicious family classic, but now gluten-free. This hearty meat-and-potatoes meal is perfect for frosty winter months, with a stick-to-your-ribs goodness that will keep you full long past dinner. Plus, it's almost as easy to prepare as it is to devour.

1. Preheat the oven to 400°F.

2. Peel the potatoes. Poke the potatoes all over with a fork, and place them on a microwave-safe plate. Microwave for 16 minutes, flipping halfway through.

3. In a Dutch oven or large oven-safe skillet, melt 1 tablespoon of butter over medium heat. Add the onion and garlic and cook until golden and fragrant, about 3 minutes. Add the beef, carrots, and thyme and cook until the beef is browned, about 5 minutes.

4. Add the corn and peas and cook until the peas are warm and tender, about 3 minutes. Drain any grease. Remove from the heat, keeping everything in the pot.

5. Cool until the potatoes are warm to the touch, about 5 minutes. Slice in half and place into a large bowl. Add the sour cream and remaining 4 tablespoons of butter.

CONTINUED

6. Using a potato masher or hand mixer on medium speed, mash the potatoes until smooth. Spread the potatoes in an even layer on top of the beef in the pot.

7. Bake for 20 minutes, then broil for an additional 2 to 3 minutes, until the potatoes become golden at their peaks. Cool for 5 minutes.

8. Store leftovers in an airtight container in the refrigerator for up to 3 days.

PRO TIP: When serving this dish to guests, sprinkle fresh thyme over the top for a fancy look.

LASAGNA FOR A CROWD

{ SERVES 10 TO 12 }

NF

PREP TIME: 15 minutes

COOK TIME: 55 minutes

8 ounces gluten-free
lasagna noodles

1½ pounds ground beef

1 medium sweet onion, diced

1 teaspoon dried onion flakes

5 cups Spaghetti Sauce (page 173)

1 (15-ounce) container
ricotta cheese

2½ cups shredded
mozzarella cheese

1 cup shredded Parmesan cheese

1½ teaspoons Italian seasoning

¼ cup chopped fresh basil,
for garnish

About once a year, my mom makes her homemade lasagna from scratch. Don't tell her, but I'm sharing the secret family recipe with you. From the homemade spaghetti sauce to the cheese and herb mix that reaches through each layer, Momma got every inch of this recipe right. Want in on another secret? There's no need to be tidy—the messier the layers, the better the lasagna tastes. At least that's what she would say.

1. Preheat the oven to 425°F. Spray a 9-by-13-inch baking dish with gluten-free cooking spray.

2. Put the lasagna noodles in a large bowl of hot water to soak.

3. In a large skillet, combine the beef, onion, and onion flakes and cook, stirring occasionally, over medium heat until browned, about 5 minutes. Drain the grease and add the spaghetti sauce. Mix to combine.

4. In a large bowl, combine the ricotta, mozzarella, and Parmesan cheese with the Italian seasoning. Mix well.

5. Spread 1 cup of spaghetti sauce on the bottom of the baking dish, then layer with lasagna

CONTINUED ◞

sheets, laying them side by side. Top the sheets with one-third of the cheese mixture, using a spatula to spread the mixture evenly. Layer on half the beef mixture, distributing as equally as possible. Repeat the layers twice so there are 3 layers total, ending in a cheese layer on top.

6. Cover with aluminum foil and bake for 45 minutes. Remove the foil and cook for an additional 10 minutes, until the edges turn golden brown and the sauce is bubbling.

7. Cool for 10 to 15 minutes, then sprinkle with basil and serve.

8. Store leftovers in an airtight container in the refrigerator for up to 5 days.

PRO TIP: Need to save time? Use no-cook gluten-free noodles, like Barilla brand.

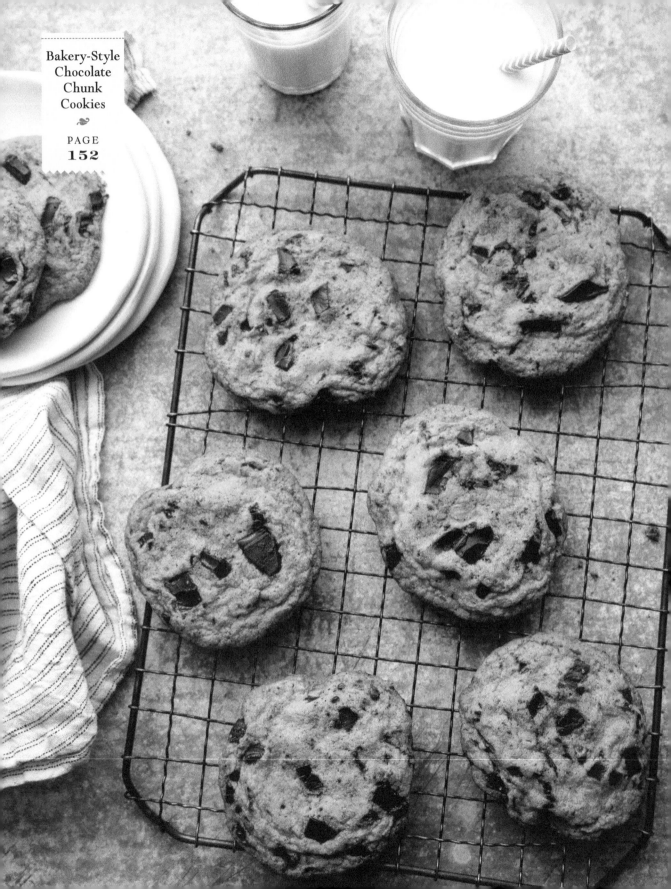

Bakery-Style
Chocolate
Chunk
Cookies

PAGE
152

{ 08 }
DESSERTS

THIN MINT COOKIES

{ MAKES 60 COOKIES }

PREP TIME: 15 minutes,
plus 35 minutes to chill

COOK TIME: 10 minutes

1 cup All-Purpose Flour Blend
(page 171), plus more for dusting

½ cup unsweetened cocoa powder

½ teaspoon baking powder

½ teaspoon baking soda

¼ teaspoon salt

5 tablespoons unsalted butter,
room temperature

¾ cup sugar

1 large egg, room temperature, and
1 large egg yolk, room temperature

1 teaspoon gluten-free
vanilla extract

2 teaspoons peppermint
extract, divided

18 ounces milk chocolate or
semisweet chocolate chips

One of the biggest challenges gluten-free folks face is the relentless craving for Girl Scout cookies every spring. It's not fair that we can't eat those delicious treats. They are everywhere you look, and there's no way to satisfy that urge to eat a batch—unless you make them yourself. These thin mint cookies are the real deal: crispy, crunchy mint-chocolate cookies smothered in mint-chocolate coating. Every bite is just as tasty as the original.

1. In a large bowl, combine the flour blend, cocoa powder, baking powder, baking soda, and salt. Mix to combine.

2. In a medium bowl, use a hand mixer on medium speed to beat the butter and sugar until well combined and smooth, 1 to 3 minutes. Add the egg and mix well. Add the egg yolk and mix well again. Beat in the vanilla and 1½ teaspoons peppermint extract, 1 to 2 minutes, until completely combined.

3. Reduce the speed to low and beat the flour mixture into the wet ingredients. Once fully combined, the dough will be very thick and sticky.

4. Roll the dough into a large ball, wrap loosely with plastic wrap, flatten, and refrigerate for 20 to 30 minutes, or up to overnight.

5. On a clean, floured surface, roll out the dough to a large circle, about ⅛ inch thick. Using a flour-dipped cookie cutter or the top of a small cup, cut the dough into 1½-inch circular cookies. Place the cookies on baking sheets lined with parchment paper. Refrigerate for an additional 15 to 30 minutes.

6. Preheat the oven to 350°F. Bake for 10 to 15 minutes, rotating the baking sheet 180 degrees halfway through, so the cookies bake evenly. Cool completely.

7. In a medium microwave-safe bowl, heat the chocolate chips on high in 30-second increments, stirring in between, until melted. Add the remaining ½ teaspoon peppermint extract and mix thoroughly.

8. Dip each cookie into the mint chocolate, using a fork to flip and coat each cookie completely. Let the excess chocolate drip off, and scrape the bottom of each cookie with another fork before setting the cookie on a fresh piece of parchment paper to harden. Let the cookies cool and harden before serving.

9. Store leftovers in an airtight container in the refrigerator for up to 1 week.

PRO TIP: If the finished cookies don't completely harden while at room temperature, place them in the refrigerator for a quick blast of cool air.

SOUTHERN PRALINES

{ MAKES 24 SAND DOLLAR–SIZE PRALINES }

VT

PREP TIME: 10 minutes

COOK TIME: 25 minutes

1 cup packed light brown sugar

1 cup granulated sugar

½ cup heavy (whipping) cream

2 tablespoons unsalted
butter, softened

1 cup pecans

1 teaspoon gluten-free
vanilla extract

Coarse sea salt, for garnish

PRO TIP: If you want more of
a praline versus a caramel, after
adding the pecans and vanilla
extract, stir continuously until the
mixture is somewhat thickened and
creamy, but has not entirely lost its
gloss, 1 to 3 minutes. Then proceed
to dropping large spoonfuls onto
the parchment paper. This adds
more air to the mixture so it's
lighter and less caramel-y.

A Southern delicacy, this finger food dessert
can't quite decide if it's a candy or a caramel.
Pralines are a melted blend of brown sugar and
butter that's sprinkled with pecans and sea salt
and then cooled. The perfect sweet treat on hot
sunny days, they won't melt in your hands, but
every sugary bite will melt in your mouth.

1. Lay a large piece of parchment paper on a
   flat surface.

2. In a large heavy saucepan over medium-high
   heat, combine the brown sugar, granulated
   sugar, cream, and butter.

3. Stirring constantly, cook until the mixture
   reaches the "soft ball" stage (238 to 240°F
   on a candy thermometer), 20 to 25 minutes.
   Immediately remove from the heat. Add the
   pecans and vanilla. Stir together.

4. Working quickly, drop large spoonfuls 2 inches
   apart onto the parchment paper. Garnish
   with sea salt. Cool to room temperature
   before serving.

5. Store leftovers in an airtight container at room
   temperature for up to 5 days.

5-INGREDIENT PEANUT BUTTER COOKIES

{ MAKES 18 COOKIES }

  DF   VT   30

PREP TIME: 10 minutes

COOK TIME: 10 minutes

1 cup all-natural peanut butter (smooth or chunky)

1 cup sugar

½ cup All-Purpose Flour Blend (page 171)

1 large egg, beaten

1 teaspoon baking soda

Want deliciously sweet peanut butter cookies in 20 minutes using only 5 ingredients? I thought you would. These cookies are crisp on the edges, but still nicely tender and moist in the center. So what are you waiting for? There are only a few minutes and a handful of ingredients between you and these amazing cookies.

1. Preheat the oven to 350°F. Line a baking sheet with parchment paper.

2. In a large bowl, mix together the peanut butter, sugar, flour blend, egg, and baking soda to form a dough. Scoop the dough into 1-inch balls and place them 3 inches apart on the parchment.

3. Bake for 9 to 11 minutes, or until the edges just start to turn golden brown. Cool on the pan for 5 minutes before transferring to a cooling rack to cool completely.

4. Store leftovers in an airtight container at room temperature for up to 5 days.

PRO TIP: Don't let these cookies cook for too long; they will harden a bit once out of the oven. Remove as soon as the outer edges start to turn golden brown.

BAKERY-STYLE CHOCOLATE CHUNK COOKIES

{ MAKES 12 COOKIES }

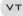

NF   VT

PREP TIME: 15 minutes,
plus 1 hour to chill

COOK TIME: 15 minutes

½ cup (1 stick) unsalted
butter, melted

½ cup packed light brown sugar

⅓ cup granulated sugar

1 large egg

1½ teaspoons gluten-free
vanilla extract

1⅓ cups All-Purpose Flour Blend
(page 171)

¼ cup potato starch (not
potato flour)

½ teaspoon baking soda

½ teaspoon salt

1⅓ cups chocolate chunks

Have you ever walked past a bakery counter with huge, perfectly chewy chocolate chip cookies coming out of the oven, the aroma of chocolate making you swoon, but all the while thinking, *I can't have that?* Yeah, been there. But now you can make them right in your own home.

1. In a large bowl, use a hand mixer on medium speed to mix the butter, brown sugar, granulated sugar, egg, and vanilla until smooth.

2. In a medium bowl, mix the flour, potato starch, baking soda, and salt. Pour one-third of the flour mixture into the bowl with the wet ingredients and mix on medium speed until smooth. Repeat twice with the remaining flour mix until a smooth dough forms, then add the chocolate chunks and use a rubber spatula to fold them in. Cover the bowl with plastic wrap and refrigerate for 1 hour. In the last 10 minutes of chilling, preheat the oven to 350°F and line a baking sheet with parchment paper.

3. Split the dough in half. Place one half back in the bowl, cover, and return to the refrigerator.

4. Split the other half into six equal parts, rolling each in your hands to form a ball. Place the balls on the lined baking sheet, leaving plenty of space between each. Bake for 14 to 16 minutes, or until the edges are golden and the centers have risen and are glistening. Cool on the baking sheet for 5 to 7 minutes before transferring to a cooling rack. Repeat step 4 for the other half of the cookie dough.

5. Store leftovers in an airtight container at room temperature for up to 5 days or freeze in a freezer-safe bag for up to 2 months.

PRO TIP: For an even more bakery-style feel to the cookies, mix up the chocolate. Combine dark chocolate chunks with semisweet or milk chocolate chips.

SOUTHERN BANANA PUDDING

{ SERVES 12 }

NF VT

PREP TIME: 20 minutes

1 (5-ounce) package gluten-free vanilla pudding mix

2 cups milk

1 package (8-ounce) cream cheese, softened

1 (14-ounce) can sweetened condensed milk

5 cups Vanilla Whipped Cream (page 169), divided

6 cups crushed Crunchy Graham Crackers (page 42), a bit reserved for garnish

1 cup sugar

1 cup unsalted butter, melted

4 bananas, sliced

PRO TIP: Be sure to use sweetened condensed milk and not evaporated milk. The cans usually look quite similar, but they produce very different results.

This banana pudding is the best dessert for someone feeling homesick. This creamy, fluffy, no-bake pudding gives you all the feels of when you were young. Of course, we have to ramp up the wow factor, so this recipe includes banana slices and a crisp cookie crust between layers of good-for-your-soul banana pudding.

1. In a large bowl, stir the pudding mix and milk together. Add the cream cheese and condensed milk. Using a hand mixer on medium speed, mix until smooth. Add 2 cups of whipped cream and whip until smooth.

2. In a medium bowl, combine the graham crackers, sugar, and butter and mix well. Spread half the mixture in the bottom of a 9-by-13-inch baking pan. Place half the sliced bananas on top of the cookie crust in an even layer, then pour half the pudding mixture on top of the bananas.

3. Repeat these three layers once more, ending with the pudding mixture.

4. Top with the remaining 3 cups of whipped cream and the remaining graham cracker crumbles. Cover with plastic wrap and refrigerate until ready to serve.

5. Store leftovers in an airtight container in the refrigerator for up to 5 days.

CARROT CAKE CUPCAKES

{ MAKES 12 CUPCAKES }

VT

PREP TIME: 15 minutes

COOK TIME: 20 minutes

1 cup almond flour

1 cup coconut flour

2 tablespoons xanthan gum

1 tablespoon baking powder

½ tablespoon baking soda

1 teaspoon ground cinnamon

1 cup sugar

¾ cup cooking oil, such as vegetable, canola, or corn

3 tablespoons unsalted butter

2 large eggs

½ cup water

1 tablespoon gluten-free vanilla extract

3 cups finely grated carrots

PRO TIP: Fill the muffin cups to the brim, as these cupcakes don't rise much while baking.

It can be hard to find a gluten-free carrot cake that isn't dry and bland—until now. This recipe is very simple and makes incredibly moist cupcakes with a golden crust. I like to frost them with Vanilla Whipped Cream (page 169).

1. Preheat the oven to 350°F. Line a 12-cup muffin tin with muffin liners or spray with gluten-free cooking spray.

2. In a medium bowl, combine the almond flour, coconut flour, xanthan gum, baking powder, baking soda, and cinnamon. Mix well.

3. In a large bowl, combine the sugar, oil, butter, eggs, water, and vanilla. Add the carrots and stir well.

4. Slowly add the dry ingredients to the large bowl. Use a hand mixer on low speed to blend the ingredients together, about 1 minute.

5. Scoop the mixture equally into the muffin cups and bake for 20 to 22 minutes, or until the tops are golden brown and a toothpick inserted into the center of a cupcake comes out clean.

6. Let cool completely before frosting.

7. Store leftovers in an airtight container at room temperature for up to 3 days.

QUICK STRAWBERRY SHORTCAKE

{ SERVES 2 }

  DF VT 30

PREP TIME: 10 minutes

COOK TIME: 1 minute

2 tablespoons coconut flour

2 tablespoons almond flour

1 tablespoon coconut sugar or granulated sugar

½ teaspoon baking powder

Pinch salt

¼ cup plain almond milk

1 large egg, beaten

¼ teaspoon strawberry extract

1 cup sliced strawberries, for garnish

Vanilla Whipped Cream (page 169), for garnish

This perfect-for-spring recipe serves up soft, fluffy strawberry-flavored cakes topped with freshly cut strawberries for a flavor-packed dessert that literally bakes in 1 minute.

1. In a medium bowl, combine the coconut flour, almond flour, sugar, baking powder, and salt. Mix well.

2. Add the almond milk, egg, and strawberry extract. Mix well, then let sit for 5 minutes to thicken.

3. Pour the dough into 1 or 2 coffee mugs (depending on their size) and microwave, one at a time, on full power for 1 minute.

4. Let sit for 5 minutes. Serve warm with sliced strawberries and whipped cream on top.

5. Store leftovers in an airtight container in the refrigerator for up to 3 days.

PRO TIP: Use the remaining strawberry extract to flavor icing, ice cream, whipped cream, smoothies, and even cheesecake.

APPLE CRUMBLE

{ SERVES 8 }

PREP TIME: 15 minutes

COOK TIME: 30 minutes

FOR THE FRUIT FILLING

4 cups fresh apples (Gala, Golden Delicious, or Red Delicious), sliced

⅓ cup granulated sugar

⅓ cup packed light brown sugar

3 tablespoons cornstarch

1 tablespoon freshly squeezed lemon juice

1 teaspoon gluten-free vanilla extract

Pinch salt

FOR THE CRUMBLE TOPPING

¾ cup gluten-free oats

½ cup almond flour

⅓ cup (5⅓ tablespoons) unsalted butter, melted

⅓ cup packed light brown sugar

½ teaspoon ground cinnamon

PRO TIP: Any of your favorite fruits or even a combination would work great in this recipe. Simply substitute the apples for pears, strawberries, blackberries, or peaches—whatever's in season.

Crumbles are a great dessert for those who don't want to do a lot of detail work but still want a delicious outcome. Just mix together the apples, pour them into a baking dish, and top them. This dish is perfect paired with ice cream or homemade Vanilla Whipped Cream (page 169) and a drizzle of fresh honey.

1. Preheat the oven to 350°F. Spray a 9-inch square baking dish or equivalent with gluten-free cooking spray.

2. **To make the fruit filling:** In a large bowl, combine the apples, granulated sugar, brown sugar, cornstarch, lemon juice, vanilla, and salt and mix well.

3. **To make the crumble topping:** In a large bowl, combine the oats, almond flour, butter, brown sugar, and cinnamon and mix well.

4. Spread the fruit evenly filling in the bottom of the baking dish. Spread the crumble topping evenly on top. Bake for 30 to 35 minutes, or until bubbling and golden brown around the edges.

5. Cool for 5 minutes and serve warm.

6. Store leftovers in an airtight container in the refrigerator for up to 3 days.

PEACH COBBLER

{ SERVES 8 }

NF VT

PREP TIME: 20 minutes

COOK TIME: 40 minutes

6 cups sliced peaches (about 2 pounds fresh peaches)

1 cup granulated sugar, divided, plus more for sprinkling

1½ cups All-Purpose Flour Blend (page 171)

2 tablespoons cornstarch

½ cup packed light brown sugar

2 teaspoons baking powder

¼ teaspoon salt

6 tablespoons cold unsalted butter, cut into small cubes

¾ cup heavy (whipping) cream

PRO TIP: Top the cobbler with fresh homemade Vanilla Whipped Cream (page 169) and a drizzle of honey.

This peach cobbler features fresh peach slices warmed beneath a layer of gooey, cookie-like dough, all the extra nooks and crannies filled with a delicious sweet sauce. Just like the cobbler Momma used to make.

1. Preheat the oven to 325°F. Spray a 9-inch square pan with gluten-free cooking spray.

2. In a large bowl, combine the peaches and ½ cup of granulated sugar.

3. In another bowl, combine the flour blend, remaining ½ cup of granulated sugar, cornstarch, brown sugar, baking powder, and salt and mix to blend. Cut in the cold butter with the back of a fork and mix until the mixture has a crumbly consistency. Stir in the cream.

4. Spread the peach mixture into the bottom of the pan.

5. Drop large spoonfuls of dough on top of the peaches. Sprinkle with a little more granulated sugar.

6. Bake for 40 to 50 minutes, or until golden on top and bubbling along the sides.

7. Cool for 5 minutes and serve warm.

8. Store leftovers in an airtight container in the refrigerator for up to 3 days.

KEY LIME PIE TRIFLE

{ SERVES 12 }

NF · VT · 30

PREP TIME: 15 minutes

FOR THE GRAHAM CRACKER CRUST

3½ cups crushed Crunchy Graham Crackers (page 42)

½ cup sugar

½ cup unsalted butter, melted

FOR THE KEY LIME FILLING

1 (8-ounce) container whipped cream topping

1 (8-ounce) package cream cheese, room temperature

½ cup milk

¼ cup freshly squeezed key lime juice

PRO TIP: Key lime juice is tarter and more potent than regular lime juice. If you don't have key lime juice on hand, you can substitute 2 tablespoons of regular lime juice and 2 tablespoons of lemon juice.

A trifle is a dessert typically displayed in a clear, tall bowl, so you can see the layers—in this case, layers of sugary crisp graham crackers and hearty dollops of dreamy, creamy key lime filling. One bite delivers crunchy sweet pieces of cookie-like crunch, and the next takes you away to a tropical paradise. This recipe is the perfect combination of crunchy and soft, light and creamy, sweet and tart.

1. **To make the graham cracker crust:** In a large bowl, combine the graham crackers, sugar, and butter and mix well.

2. **To make the key lime filling:** In the bowl of a stand mixer fitted with the whisk attachment or a large bowl with a hand mixer, combine the whipped cream, cream cheese, milk, and lime juice and mix on medium speed until stiff peaks form, 5 to 7 minutes.

3. Fill the bottom of a trifle bowl or other clear serving bowl with one-third of the graham cracker mixture, followed by one-third of the key lime filling. Repeat twice, or until both mixtures are used up.

4. Cover the top of the glass container with plastic wrap and refrigerate until ready to serve.

5. Store leftovers covered with plastic wrap in the refrigerator for up to 5 days.

CLASSIC CHEESECAKE

{ SERVES 10 }

NF VT

PREP TIME: 20 minutes,
plus 4 hours to chill

FOR THE GRAHAM
CRACKER CRUST

2½ cups crushed Crunchy Graham
Crackers (page 42)

⅓ cup packed light brown sugar

10 tablespoons (1¼ sticks) unsalted
butter, melted

FOR THE CHEESECAKE
FILLING

3 (8-ounce) packages
cream cheese

½ cup granulated sugar

5 tablespoons powdered sugar

¼ cup sour cream

1½ teaspoons gluten-free
vanilla extract

1¼ cups heavy (whipping) cream

PRO TIP: Give this cheesecake
a twist by swapping the vanilla
extract for strawberry, lemon, or
other flavors of extract.

One of the comfort foods I missed most when
first going gluten-free was cheesecake—thick
and rich, with a fluffy yet dense core and a
sweet, soft crust. So I created this recipe for a
delicious no-bake cheesecake, which you can
customize with any flavor you'd like. I bet this
recipe will be one of your favorites.

1. **Make the graham cracker crust:** In a
    medium bowl, mix together the graham
    crackers, brown sugar, and butter and place
    the mixture in the bottom of a springform
    pan. Press down firmly so it doesn't fall apart
    when serving. Place the crust in the freezer
    while making the cheesecake filling, 10 to
    15 minutes.

2. **Make the cheesecake filling:** In the bowl of a
    stand mixer fitted with the whisk attachment
    or a large bowl with a hand mixer on medium
    speed, whip the cream cheese, granulated
    sugar, powdered sugar, sour cream, and vanilla
    until well blended and smooth, 3 to 4 minutes.

3. Pour in the cream and whip the mixture
    on medium speed until stiff peaks form,
    3 to 5 minutes. Scrape the filling into the
    crust-lined pan, spreading evenly.

4. Cover and refrigerate for 4 to 6 hours
    before serving.

5. Store leftovers in an airtight container in the
    refrigerator for up to 5 days.

PUMPKIN PECAN BREAD PUDDING

{ SERVES 10 }

VT

PREP TIME: 10 minutes

COOK TIME: 55 minutes

7 cups cubed day-old Sandwich Bread (page 50)

1 cup heavy (whipping) cream

1 cup pumpkin puree

4 large eggs

½ cup chopped pecans

½ cup butterscotch chips

½ cup packed light brown sugar

½ cup unsalted butter, melted

1½ teaspoons gluten-free vanilla extract

1½ teaspoons pumpkin pie spice, plus more for sprinkling

PRO TIP: Homemade Vanilla Whipped Cream (page 169) and gluten-free caramel sauce or honey make great garnishes for this dish.

This pumpkin pecan bread pudding is the perfect dessert when you don't want to lift more than a finger or two. Sweet chunks of toasted bread smothered in a sticky sauce will make anyone's day better. Plus, this gooey pumpkin treat uses up extra gluten-free bread you may have lying around.

1. Preheat the oven to 225°F. Spray the inside of a Dutch oven or large oven-safe pot with gluten-free cooking spray.

2. Place the bread cubes in the bottom of the pot.

3. In a large bowl, combine the cream, pumpkin puree, eggs, pecans, butterscotch chips, brown sugar, butter, vanilla, and pumpkin pie spice and stir until well combined.

4. Pour the mixture over the bread cubes and stir until just combined. Sprinkle with a little more pumpkin pie spice.

5. Cover and cook on low for 55 to 60 minutes, until warm, moist, and gooey. Remove from the heat and serve warm.

6. Store leftovers in an airtight container in the refrigerator for up to 3 days.

MISSISSIPPI MUD BARS

{ MAKES 12 TO 16 BARS }

PREP TIME: 15 minutes, plus 30 minutes to chill

FOR THE PEANUT BUTTER CRUST

2 cups peanut butter

1½ cups packed light brown sugar

1½ cups powdered sugar

6 tablespoons unsalted butter, melted

FOR THE MISSISSIPPI MUD TOPPING

3¼ cups chocolate chips

1½ cups gluten-free mini marshmallows

½ cup coarsely chopped pecans

Pinch coarse sea salt

PRO TIP: Once firm, these squares are fine stored at room temperature, but something about chilled Mississippi Mud Bars hits your taste buds just right.

Chocolate, marshmallows, and peanut butter—the perfect blend for your sugar craving. Don't forget to balance out the sweetness with a sprinkle of sea salt.

1. Line a 9-inch square pan with parchment paper.

2. **To make the peanut butter crust:** In a medium bowl, stir together the peanut butter, brown sugar, powdered sugar, and butter until well blended. Press evenly into the bottom of the pan.

3. **To make the Mississippi mud topping:** In a medium microwave-safe bowl, microwave the chocolate chips on high in 30-second increments, stirring in between, until melted. Pour half the melted chocolate over the peanut butter crust and spread evenly.

4. Sprinkle the marshmallows and nuts over the melted chocolate layer, then drizzle the remaining melted chocolate on top. Sprinkle with a pinch or two of sea salt.

5. Refrigerate until firm, 2 to 3 hours, or freeze for 30 to 60 minutes. Cut into squares and serve.

CHOCOLATE MOUSSE

{ SERVES 6 TO 8 }

PREP TIME: 15 minutes,
plus 1 hour to chill

COOK TIME: 5 minutes

8 ounces milk or dark baking
chocolate, coarsely chopped

2 cups heavy (whipping)
cream, divided

2 tablespoons powdered sugar
(optional, see pro tip)

1½ teaspoons gluten-free
vanilla extract

PRO TIP: If you use milk chocolate
for the mousse, you may not need
to add the powdered sugar. Taste
the mixture before adding the
powdered sugar to determine
whether it's already sweet enough.

A decadent chocolate dessert that's as fluffy as
air and won't weigh you down? That's what this
recipe's all about. Sweet pieces of your favorite
chocolate bar are melted into whipping cream
and then beaten to light and airy perfection.
While it may taste like you've been slaving
away for hours to perfect this dish, it couldn't
be easier.

1. Place the chocolate in a large heatproof bowl.

2. In a small saucepan, heat 1 cup of cream over
    medium heat just until it starts to simmer
    around the edges.

3. Pour the simmering cream into the bowl with
    the chopped chocolate. Stir until the chocolate
    has fully melted. Add the powdered sugar
    and vanilla. Stir continuously while adding in
    the remaining 1 cup of cream. Stir until well
    combined and smooth.

4. Cover and refrigerate for 1 to 2 hours. Remove
    from the refrigerator, scrape the chocolate
    mixture into the bowl of a stand mixer fitted
    with the whisk attachment or a large bowl with
    a hand mixer, and mix on medium until stiff
    peaks form, 1 to 2 minutes. Serve immediately

5. Store leftovers in an airtight container in the
    refrigerator for up to 5 days.

FLOURLESS CHOCOLATE TORTE
{ SERVES 12 }

NF VT

PREP TIME: 20 minutes,
plus 1 hour to chill

COOK TIME: 30 minutes

1¼ cups (2½ sticks) salted
butter, divided

14 ounces bittersweet chocolate
chips, divided

1½ cups sugar

6 large eggs

1 cup unsweetened cocoa powder

1½ cups berries of choice

This chocolate torte is one of my all-time favorite
desserts. Not only is it scrumptious, but it's also
incredibly easy to make and tastes like a gourmet
chef prepared it. This moist, rich chocolate
torte is topped with a creamy chocolate coating,
and the fresh berries melted into the top make
it look absolutely divine. Keep it chilled in the
refrigerator to make every bite that much better.

1. Preheat the oven to 375°F and spray a
   9-inch oven-safe pie plate with gluten-free
   cooking spray.

2. Fill a large saucepan two-thirds full of water
   and bring to a boil. Place a medium saucepan
   over the large saucepan to create a double
   boiler. Inside the medium saucepan, place
   1 cup (2 sticks) of butter and 8 ounces of
   chocolate chips. Stir until melted.

3. Remove the medium saucepan from the heat,
   add the sugar, and stir until well blended. Add
   the eggs and beat well. Add the cocoa powder
   and stir until blended and smooth.

4. Pour the batter into the pie plate and bake for
   22 to 24 minutes, or until the edges are cooked
   but the center is still jiggly and moist. Cool for
   15 minutes. Carefully invert the pie plate to
   release the torte and transfer it right-side up
   onto a serving platter to cool further.

5. In a small microwave-safe bowl, combine the remaining
    4 tablespoons of butter and remaining 6 ounces of chocolate chips.
    Microwave on high in 30-second increments, stirring in between,
    until the butter and chocolate have melted into a blended sauce.
    Immediately pour the chocolate sauce on top of the cooled torte,
    using the back of a spoon or a spatula to spread it evenly on top.
    Working quickly, place the berries on top of the chocolate. Allow
    to set for 1 hour before cutting into slices and serving.

6. Store leftovers in an airtight container in the refrigerator for up to
    1 week or in a freezer-safe bag in the freezer for up to 2 months.

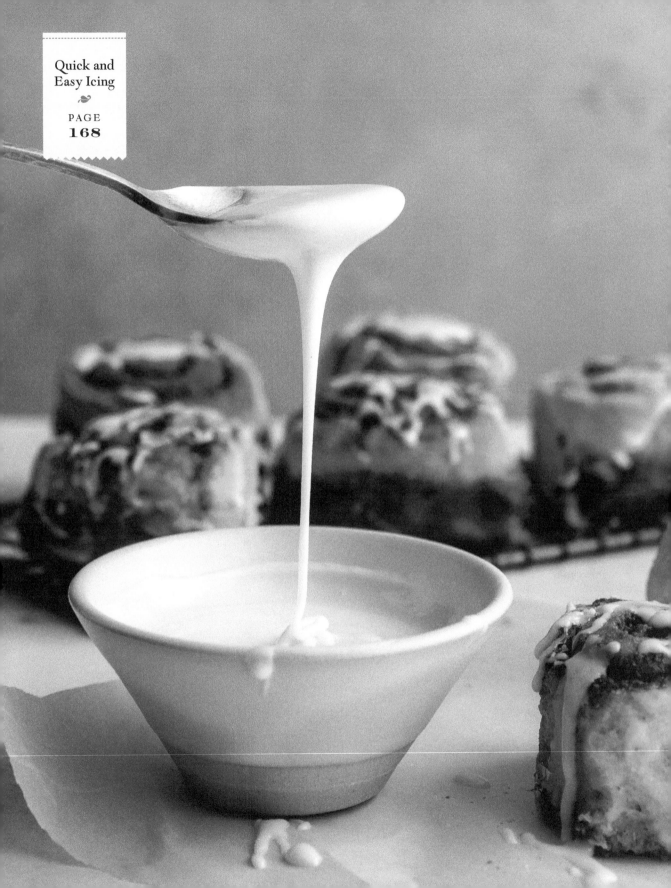

Quick and
Easy Icing

PAGE
168

{ 09 }

GLUTEN-FREE STAPLES

QUICK AND EASY ICING

{ MAKES ABOUT ½ CUP }

PREP TIME: 5 minutes

1½ cups powdered sugar

3 tablespoons milk

This vanilla icing is perfect drizzled over your favorite desserts and breakfast sweets. Try it on Overnight French Toast Casserole (page 29), Sweet Quinoa Breakfast Bars (page 16), Grandma's Old-Fashioned Baked Donuts (page 25), Carrot Cake Cupcakes (page 155), or Apple Crumble (page 157).

1. In a medium bowl, combine the sugar and milk and stir well until smooth and creamy.

2. Drizzle over anything.

3. Store in an airtight container in the refrigerator for up to 3 days.

PRO TIP: If you like a thicker icing, reduce the milk by ½ tablespoon. If you'd like to thin it out, stir in ½ to 1 tablespoon of extra milk. For a flavored icing, add in ½ teaspoon of vanilla, strawberry, almond, or lemon extract.

VANILLA WHIPPED CREAM

{ MAKES ABOUT 1 CUP }

PREP TIME: 10 minutes, plus 20 minutes to chill

1 (13.5-ounce) can full-fat coconut milk, chilled

1½ teaspoons gluten-free vanilla extract

This coconut whipped cream is so incredibly easy to make and great for those with dairy sensitivities. It's every bit as sweet and creamy as traditional whipped cream, with an extra touch of freshness. It's the perfect topping for all your favorite desserts (see pro tip). You can even use it as frosting.

1. Put the coconut milk and a large glass or metal bowl in the refrigerator and chill until cold, about 20 minutes.

2. Turn the can of cold coconut milk upside down so the liquid portion is at the top. Discard the liquids, or save for another recipe.

3. Pour the coconut milk solids into the chilled bowl. Using a hand mixer on medium speed, beat until it begins to thicken, about 5 minutes.

4. Add the vanilla and continue to beat until the mixture reaches your desired thickness, about 2 more minutes.

5. Store in an airtight container in the refrigerator for up to 1 day.

PRO TIP: For a sweet garnish, dollop this delicious cream over fresh fruit or Southern Banana Pudding (page 154), Quick Strawberry Shortcake (page 156), Peach Cobbler (page 158), Key Lime Pie Trifle (page 159), or Chocolate Mousse (page 163).

BREAD CRUMBS

{ MAKES ABOUT 5 CUPS }

DF   NF   V   30

PREP TIME: 5 minutes

COOK TIME: 15 minutes

1 loaf Sandwich Bread (page 50)
or other gluten-free bread, cut into
large cubes

3 tablespoons Italian seasoning

These bread crumbs are used in many recipes throughout this book, but don't let that limit you. Use these perfectly golden, savory bread crumbs to add flavor and a tasty crunch to just about any dish. The top of your next casserole is calling.

1. Preheat the oven to 350°F and spray a rimmed baking sheet with gluten-free cooking spray.

2. Place the bread in a food processor and process until it turns to crumbs the size of grated Parmesan cheese.

3. Spread in an even layer on the baking sheet. Sprinkle with the Italian seasoning, stir, and spray with a light coating of gluten-free cooking spray.

4. Bake for 15 minutes, stirring every 5 minutes, until golden and fragrant.

5. Cool completely.

6. Store in an airtight container at room temperature or in the freezer for up to 6 months.

PRO TIP: Make 2 or 3 batches of this recipe at a time and freeze the extra in small portions. When it's time to use it, you can pull out the exact amount for any recipe straight from the freezer. No need to defrost.

ALL-PURPOSE FLOUR BLEND

{ MAKES 2¼ CUPS }

DF · NF · V · 30

PREP TIME: 3 minutes

1 cup brown rice flour

½ cup white rice flour

½ cup potato starch (not potato flour)

¼ cup tapioca flour

2 teaspoons xanthan gum

What could be better than an all-purpose gluten-free flour you can use in all sorts of dishes? You'll always want to have this blend on hand. Try this flour blend any time you need all-purpose flour, including in Breakfast Beignets (page 20), Grandma's Old-Fashioned Baked Donuts (page 25), Ooey Gooey Cinnamon Rolls (page 27), Crispy Cheese Crackers (page 43), Thin Pizza Crust (page 44), Sandwich Bread (page 50), and Savory Potato Rolls (page 52), to name a few.

In a large bowl, combine the brown rice flour, white rice flour, potato starch, tapioca flour, and xanthan gum and mix well. Store in an airtight container at room temperature for up to 2 months.

PRO TIP: I highly recommend Bob's Red Mill Potato Starch. It's affordable and usually easy to find. Potato starch is in the baking aisle near the flours in many large grocery stores, in health food stores, and online.

BISCUIT MIX

{ MAKES ABOUT 5 CUPS }

PREP TIME: 5 minutes

2 cups white rice flour

1¼ cups coconut flour

1 cup milk powder

½ cup cornstarch

¼ cup sugar

2 teaspoons baking powder

1 teaspoon baking soda

½ teaspoon salt

Just like the boxed variety, this biscuit mix combines a few simple ingredients to make the base for tons of baked goods. You'll see it in Classic Waffles (page 23), Easy Fluffy Pancakes (page 22), Zucchini Bread (page 53), and Mini Buttermilk Biscuits (page 56).

Combine the white rice flour, coconut flour, milk powder, cornstarch, sugar, baking powder, baking soda, and salt in a large mixing bowl and stir thoroughly to combine. Store in an airtight glass container at room temperature for up to 2 months.

PRO TIP: I have found that biscuit mix stored in airtight glass containers, like Mason jars, tends to stay fresher longer.

SPAGHETTI SAUCE

{ MAKES 5 CUPS }

 NF VT 30

PREP TIME: 5 minutes

COOK TIME: 20 minutes

3 cups water

2 (6-ounce) cans tomato paste

3 dried bay leaves

3 tablespoons grated
Parmesan cheese

3 tablespoons dried oregano

1½ tablespoons dried onion flakes

2 teaspoons sugar

1 teaspoon minced garlic

½ teaspoon garlic salt

½ teaspoon freshly ground
black pepper

Did you know that gluten is sometimes used as a stabilizer in spaghetti sauce? Bottled gluten-free pasta sauce is fine in a pinch, but this homemade sauce is a savory marinara you can use in nearly any Italian dish. A simple simmer is the only thing that stands between you and your new favorite sauce.

1. In a large pot or Dutch oven over medium heat, combine the water, tomato paste, bay leaves, Parmesan cheese, oregano, onion flakes, sugar, garlic, garlic salt, and pepper and stir well.

2. Simmer for 20 minutes for the flavors to come together. Cool for 2 to 3 minutes before serving.

3. Store in an airtight container in the refrigerator for up to 5 days, or in the freezer for up to 4 months.

PRO TIP: Use this sauce in dishes like Marinara Meatballs (page 135), Pepperoni Pizza (page 114), Chicken Parmesan (page 121), and Lasagna for a Crowd (page 143).

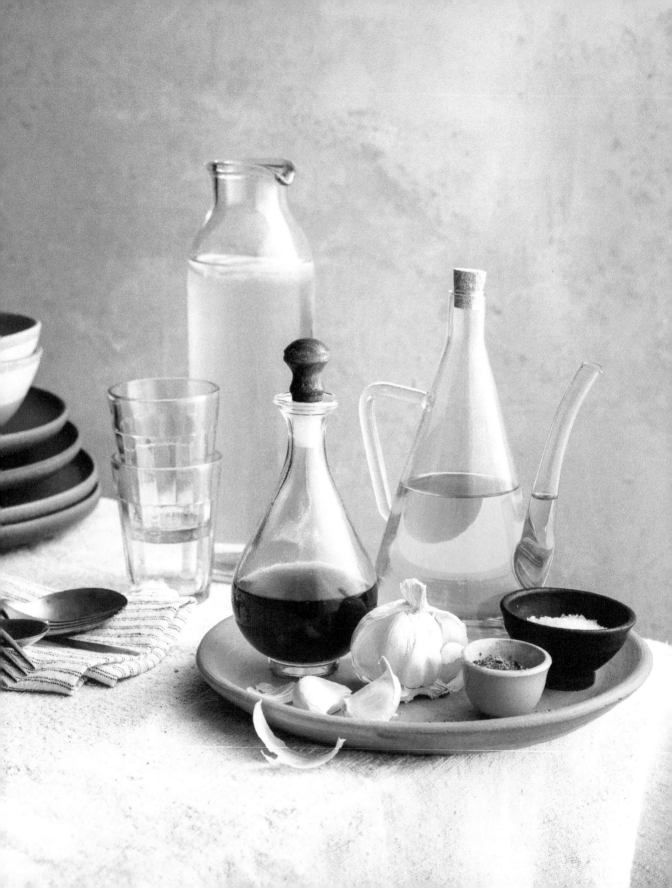

MEASUREMENT CONVERSIONS

VOLUME EQUIVALENTS (LIQUID)

US Standard	US Standard (ounces)	Metric (approximate)
2 tablespoons	1 fl. oz.	30 mL
¼ cup	2 fl. oz.	60 mL
½ cup	4 fl. oz.	120 mL
1 cup	8 fl. oz.	240 mL
1½ cups	12 fl. oz.	355 mL
2 cups or 1 pint	16 fl. oz.	475 mL
4 cups or 1 quart	32 fl. oz.	1 L
1 gallon	128 fl. oz.	4 L

OVEN TEMPERATURES

Fahrenheit (F)	Celsius (C) (approximate)
250°F	120°C
300°F	150°C
325°F	165°C
350°F	180°C
375°F	190°C
400°F	200°C
425°F	220°C
450°F	230°C

VOLUME EQUIVALENTS (DRY)

US Standard	Metric (approximate)
⅛ teaspoon	0.5 mL
¼ teaspoon	1 mL
½ teaspoon	2 mL
¾ teaspoon	4 mL
1 teaspoon	5 mL
1 tablespoon	15 mL
¼ cup	59 mL
⅓ cup	79 mL
½ cup	118 mL
⅔ cup	156 mL
¾ cup	177 mL
1 cup	235 mL
2 cups or 1 pint	475 mL
3 cups	700 mL
4 cups or 1 quart	1 L

WEIGHT EQUIVALENTS

US Standard	Metric (approximate)
½ ounce	15 g
1 ounce	30 g
2 ounces	60 g
4 ounces	115 g
8 ounces	225 g
12 ounces	340 g
16 ounces or 1 pound	455 g

RESOURCES

BlessHerHeartYall.com
If you like the recipes in this book, visit my website for hundreds of other gluten-free comfort food recipes.

Celiac.org
A great resource to find out the latest information on gluten-free diets.

GlutenFreeOnAShoestring.com
This site has lots of useful tips and recipes for the very basics needed for gluten-free baking.

SUBSTITUTIONS FOR OTHER ALLERGIES

If you're one of the unlucky folks who has additional food allergies, I feel your pain. Throughout the book I suggest replacements for dairy, but here are some other common allergens that come up in the recipes that you may want to substitute.

IF A RECIPE CALLS FOR . . .	SUBSTITUTE WITH . . .
Peanut butter	Almond butter, sunflower seed butter, or pecan butter
Eggs	Commercial egg replacers (see package directions for amount of replacer to use per egg)
Tree nuts	Roasted pumpkin seeds or sunflower seeds

INDEX

ACKNOWLEDGMENTS

I would like to thank my family and friends for their incredible support through this book-publishing process. I achieved this success only because of my loving tribe. I would like to thank Julie Kirk and Tai Anderson for their enthusiasm in their roles as research assistants, especially in the pivotal areas of taste-testing and dish-cleaning. Bless your hearts! Lastly, thank you to everyone who has read a post, shared a photo, cooked a recipe, or trusted me enough that you went out and spent your own hard-earned money on this book. I appreciate you all.

ABOUT THE AUTHOR

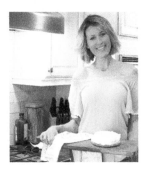 **Jessica Kirk,** DVM, is an outdoor-, food-, and wine-loving extrovert. By day, she is a veterinarian in academia. By night, she teaches others how to cook gluten-free the easy way through her website BlessHerHeartYall.com. She lives in Roswell, Georgia, with her family; two Boston terriers, Pippy and Thelma; and horse, Scuba.